Medical Statistics

Mr Paul Cool

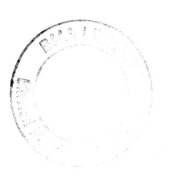

2nd Edition (reprinted) 2010

Medical Statistics
by Paul Cool

Cover Design: Louise Scott

To Karen & Oliver

Published in United Kingdom
Institute Orthopaedics
Oswestry

ISBN: 978-0-9539982-8-9

Introduction

Most postgraduate trainees do not enjoy studying statistics. However, statistics is nowadays an important part of the intercollegiate fellowship examination. It is therefore necessary to have a basic understanding of statistics. Statisticians write most books about statistics and consequently most of us non statisticians are easily confused.
Statistics is a science that cannot be learned of by heart and it is essential to have some understanding of the principles. I hope in this book to explain the most basic of these principles.

Physicists have been using mathematical models to describe the behaviour of inanimate objects. Overall, these models are very successful in predicting the behaviour of these objects (for example Newton's laws). However, when we are dealing with biological systems, models are less helpful. This is due to the great biological variety. All biological specimens of the same species are slightly different and behave differently under the same circumstances. For example, some of *Staphylococcus Aureus* bacteria die when treated with the antibiotic flucloxacillin. They are called sensitive to this antibiotic. However, there are other strains of *Staphylococcus Aureus* that are resistant to this antibiotic. Obviously, it is more difficult to predict the behaviour of *Staphylococcus Aureus* when some of the bacteria die under the influence of flucloxacillin, whilst others do not. To make matters even more complicated, some of these bacteria might become resistant to flucloxacillin during treatment.
For reasons of biological diversity, we are unable to create a mathematical model that accurately describes the behaviour of biological systems. Consequently, if we are doing an experiment with biological specimen, there is always a degree of uncertainty. The aim of medical statistics is to assess this uncertainty and state how sure we are that a statement is correct. In making statements it is therefore customary to state the degree of this uncertainty (for example $p = 0.05$; see chapter 5).

Of all chapters, chapter 2 is perhaps the most difficult to understand. This chapter explains how to calculate different probabilities. The mathematics is somewhat more complex than in the other chapters. However, a good understanding of the principles behind probabilities is essential to understand statistics. Once the reader understands these, the remainder of the book should be fairly easy to follow.

At the end of each chapter there is a summary that highlights the most important points. Most chapters have questions, the answers of which can be found at the end of the book. The questions are designed to allow the reader to practice the calculations explained.

This book is not intended to be a complete textbook of statistics. Its aim is merely to explain the most basic medical statistics and it is hoped that this is sufficient for most trainees to pass their examinations.

I would like to thank my teachers, Mr David Jaffray, Mr David Ford, Mr David Williams and Mr Rob Grimer. Every day I benefit from what they have taught me.

I am extremely grateful to Mrs Louise Scott for the design of the front cover of this book. My brother Peter Cool has been of invaluable help making some of the graphs.

Finally, profits will benefit the Orthopaedic Oncology Research Fund at the Institute of Orthopaedics in Oswestry.

Paul Cool
Oswestry
December 2003

Thank you very much for making the first edition of this book so successful. I am very grateful for all your comments. They have been incorporated in this second edition.
To make the book more durable, this second edition is now hard back bound. Also, a chapter about growth curves z-scores and t-scores has been added (chapter 4).
There has been considerable interest from non orthopaedic specialist registrars. Therefore, the title has been changed to Medical Statistics. Hopefully, this will catch a wider readership.

Paul Cool
Oswestry
December 2006

Contents

Chapter 1 - Epidemiology

When we are talking about a disease, it is important to define the disease first. The definition of disease may vary between specialties and amongst specialists in the same speciality.

For example, carpal tunnel syndrome can be diagnosed on the history, clinical examination, neurophysiological tests or a combination of these. Obviously, it is important to know what diagnostic criteria have been used in order to compare outcomes of different treatment modalities. If different definitions of disease have been used, it might not be possible to compare the different studies as it can lead to wrong conclusions.

Screening

The definition of disease may also vary according to what is required. **Screening is the application of a test to asymptomatic individuals to assess the likelihood that an individual has a particular disease**. Therefore, screening is done on large populations and the test being used should be suitable to be applied to a large number of people. It should pick up all individuals who have the disease (high sensitivity; see chapter 7). Furthermore, the test should be simple, cheap and minimally invasive. Obviously, the disease screened for should be serious enough to make subsequent treatment necessary.

Individuals with a positive test require further tests to make a definite diagnosis. For example, a heel prick blood test is being used to diagnose phenylketonuria (an autosomal recessive hereditary condition that if left untreated results in severe mental retardation). Further genetic testing after a positive screening test is required.

It is possible that an individual tested positive on the screening test, but after further testing has been show not to have the disease. This is called a false positive result and this will be discussed further in chapter 7.

Once people have been diagnosed as having the disease following a screening test, treatment should be available, otherwise there would have been no point in performing the screening in the first place! In the example above, omitting phenylalanine from the diet can treat phenylketonuria.

Surveillance

Surveillance is different than screening. **In surveillance of disease, one looks for changes in trends or distribution of the disease**. For example the influence of smoking on lung cancer.

Prevalence

Epidemiologist use prevalence and incidence as measures of how common a disease is.
Prevalence is the total number of individuals with the disease at a particular point in time divided by the population at risk. In other words, it is the proportion of the population that suffers from the disease.

Incidence

Incidence is the number of NEW cases of the disease per year divided by the population at risk. For example there are approximately 150 new cases of osteosarcoma per year in Britain. The population of Britain is approximately 50000000. Therefore the Incidence of osteosarcoma is 150 / 50000000 or 3 per million.

So when the population and the disease are stable:

$$\textbf{Prevalence = Prevalence}_{\textbf{start}} \textbf{ + Incidence * Time}$$

In trying to compare the influence of an exposure on a disease, it is obviously more useful to compare incidences rather than prevalences.

Risk factor

Patients often ask us what the *cause* of their disease is. In some cases, this is question is easy to answer. For example, a fracture is usually caused by trauma and bacteria cause infection.

However, in other cases we have difficulties in defining one particular cause for a disease. For example, we don't know the cause of arthritis. But we do know several factors that increase the risk on developing arthritis, such as age, trauma and genetic factors.

A risk factor is an exposure or attribute that increases the probability of a disease.

We will now look at an (made up) example, and examine if previous deep sea diving is a risk factor for later developing osteonecrosis of the femoral head.

Somehow, we have identified a study-group of 450 subjects over the age of 50. We question all these subjects and ask them if they have been deep-sea diving below a level of 10 metres for at least once in their lives. Furthermore, all subjects had a pelvic radiograph taken that has been scrutinised by a radiologist for signs of osteonecrosis. This is an example of a cross-sectional study (chapter 11). Here, we won't go further in the advantages and disadvantages of such a study.

In our example, we assume that 150 subjects have been deep-sea diving and 300 have not. Of the 150 subjects who have been deep-sea diving, 15 had signs of osteonecrosis on the radiographs whilst 135 did not. In the group of 300 non deep-sea divers, only 2 people had signs of osteonecrosis on the radiographs.

We can now construct a two by two table as follows:

	Disease	**No Disease**
Exposure	a	b
No Exposure	c	d

If we fill in the figures of our example:

	Disease (Osteonecrosis)	No Disease (No Osteonecrosis)
Exposure (Deep-Sea diving)	15	135
No Exposure (No Deep-Sea diving)	2	298

We can now calculate the **absolute risks** of deep-sea diving and not diving as follows:

Absolute Risk 1 $= \dfrac{a}{(a+b)}$

Absolute Risk 2 $= \dfrac{c}{(c+d)}$

Or, in our example:

Absolute Risk Deep-Sea Diving $= \dfrac{15}{(15+135)} = \dfrac{15}{150} = 0.1$

So, 1 in 10 deep-sea divers develop osteonecrosis of the femoral head.

Absolute Risk Not Diving $= \dfrac{2}{(2+298)} = \dfrac{2}{300} \approx 0.0067$

Or 1 in 150 non-divers will develop osteonecrosis of the femoral head.

Relative Risk

We can now also calculate the relative risk.
The relative risk is the risk of developing the disease that is due to an exposure in the exposed group.
In other words it is the absolute risk of developing the disease in the exposed group divided by the absolute risk of developing the disease in the non-exposed group. Or:

$$\textbf{Relative Risk} = \frac{\dfrac{a}{(a+b)}}{\dfrac{c}{(c+d)}}$$

In our example this is:

$$\textbf{Relative Risk} = \frac{\dfrac{15}{150}}{\dfrac{2}{300}} = \frac{0.1}{0.0067} \approx 14.93$$

So in our example, the risk of developing osteonecrosis of the femoral head is 15 (14.93) times higher in deep-sea divers than it is in non-divers. The absolute risk of deep sea diving was 1 in 10 (0.1). However 1 in 150 (0.0067) non-divers also developed the disease. The relative risk corrects for the occurrence of the disease in the non-exposed people.

Odds Ratio

Finally, we can define the odds ratio.
The odds ratio is the ratio of the odds of a disease occurring among exposed individuals to that of it occurring in unexposed individuals.

$$\text{Odds Ratio} = \frac{\dfrac{\dfrac{a}{(a+b)}}{\dfrac{b}{(a+b)}}}{\dfrac{\dfrac{c}{(c+d)}}{\dfrac{d}{(c+d)}}} = \frac{\dfrac{a}{(a+b)} * \dfrac{(a+b)}{b}}{\dfrac{c}{(c+d)} * \dfrac{(c+d)}{d}} = \frac{\dfrac{a}{b}}{\dfrac{c}{d}} = \frac{a*d}{b*c}$$

Or in our example:

$$\text{Odds Ratio} = \frac{15*298}{135*2} = \frac{4470}{270} \approx 16.56$$

So in this example, the odds that a person who has been deep-sea diving develops osteonecrosis of the femoral head is 16.56 times to that of a person who has not been diving.

So let us now look at three different theoretical situations:

1. **Exposure has *no effect* on incidence of disease**
   - For example blue eyes have ***no effect*** on the risk of developing arthritis
   - $a = c = 5$ & $b = d = 95$

	Disease (Arthritis)	**No Disease** (No Arthritis)
Exposure (Blue Eyes)	5	95
No Exposure (Brown eyes)	5	95

$$\text{Absolute Risk 1} = \frac{a}{(a+b)} = \frac{5}{(5+95)} = 0.05$$

$$\text{Absolute Risk 2} = \frac{c}{(c+d)} = \frac{5}{(5+95)} = 0.05$$

$$\text{Relative Risk} = \frac{\dfrac{a}{(a+b)}}{\dfrac{c}{(c+d)}} = \frac{\dfrac{5}{(5+95)}}{\dfrac{5}{(5+95)}} = 1$$

$$\text{Odds Ratio} = \frac{a*d}{b*c} = \frac{5*95}{95*5} = 1$$

2. Exposure *increases* incidence of disease

- For example smoking *increases* the risk of lung cancer
- a >> c & b << d

	Disease (Lung Ca)	**No Disease** (No Lung Ca)
Exposure (Smoking)	99	1
No Exposure (No Smoking)	1	99

$$\text{Absolute Risk 1} = \frac{a}{(a+b)} = \frac{99}{(99+1)} = 0.99$$

$$\text{Absolute Risk 2} = \frac{c}{(c+d)} = \frac{1}{(1+99)} = 0.01$$

$$\text{Relative Risk} = \frac{\dfrac{a}{(a+b)}}{\dfrac{c}{(c+d)}} = \frac{\dfrac{99}{(99+1)}}{\dfrac{1}{(1+99)}} = 99$$

$$\text{Odds Ratio} = \frac{a*d}{b*c} = \frac{99*99}{1*1} = 9801$$

3. Exposure *decreases* incidence of disease
- For example vaccination *decreases* the risk of polio
- a << c & b >> d

	Disease (Polio)	No Disease (No Polio)
Exposure (Vaccinated)	1	99
No Exposure (Not Vaccinated)	99	1

$$\text{Absolute Risk 1} = \frac{a}{(a+b)} = \frac{1}{(1+99)} = 0.01$$

$$\text{Absolute Risk 2} = \frac{c}{(c+d)} = \frac{99}{(99+1)} = 0.99$$

$$\text{Relative Risk} = \frac{\dfrac{a}{(a+b)}}{\dfrac{c}{(c+d)}} = \frac{\dfrac{1}{(1+99)}}{\dfrac{99}{(99+1)}} = \frac{1}{99} \approx 0.0101$$

$$\text{Odds Ratio} = \frac{a*d}{b*c} = \frac{1*1}{99*99} \approx 0.0001$$

So, the absolute risk is always between 0 and 1

The relative risk is always larger than 0.
If the relative risk =1, there is **no** increased risk for developing the disease.
A relative risk less than 1 (but larger than 0) indicates that the exposure protects against disease.
If the relative risk is larger than 1, there is an increased risk for developing the disease. The greater the value, the stronger the link is between exposure and disease.
In other words, if the relative risk = 1 the exposure is not a risk factor for disease. The larger the relative risk, the bigger the risk becomes. If the relative risk is very high, one could call it the **cause** of the disease. There is no cut-off point between risk factor and cause; but there is a spectrum.

Exactly the same is true for the odds ratio. If the value of the odds ratio is between 0 and 1, the exposure protects against disease. An odds ratio greater than 1 indicates that the exposure is a risk factor. The larger the odds ratio becomes, the stronger the risk of developing disease. If the odds ratio =1, the exposure has no influence of the development of disease.

Summary Chapter 1

- **Screening is the application of a test to asymptomatic individuals to assess the likelihood that an individual has a particular disease**

- **Surveillance of disease is used to look for changes in trends or distribution of the disease**

- Prevalence $= \dfrac{\text{Number of Existing Cases per Year}}{\text{Population at Risk}}$

- Incidence $= \dfrac{\text{Number of New Cases per Year}}{\text{Population at Risk}}$

- **Prevalence = Prevalence$_{\text{start}}$ + Incidence * Time**
  (when population and disorder stable)

- **A risk factor is an exposure or attribute that increases the probability of a disease**

- **The relative risk is the risk of developing the disease that is due to an exposure in the exposed group**

- **The odds ratio is the ratio of the odds of a disease occurring among exposed individuals to that of it occurring in unexposed individuals**

	Disease	No Disease
Exposure	a	b
No Exposure	c	d

- Absolute Risk 1 = $\dfrac{a}{(a+b)}$

- Absolute Risk 2 = $\dfrac{c}{(c+d)}$

- Relative Risk = $\dfrac{\dfrac{a}{(a+b)}}{\dfrac{c}{(c+d)}}$

- Odds Ratio = $\dfrac{a*d}{b*c}$

Questions Chapter 1

On 1st January 2000, there were 1000 people in Britain (population 50 million) who had osteosarcoma. During the year, 200 new cases of osteosarcoma were diagnosed and 75 patients died. Of the 75 patients who died, 50 died of disease and 25 died from other causes. The population remained stable during the year.

1. What was the prevalence on 1st January 2000?

2. What was the prevalence on 1st January 2001?

3. What is the incidence in 2000?

In a cross-sectional study, radiographs were taken of 500 wrists. A radiologist reviewed all radiographs and made a diagnosis of Kienböck's disease in 15 subjects.
To determine if negative ulnar variance was a risk factor for Kienböck's disease, all wrists were also examined for negative ulnar variance. Out of the 500 wrists, the radiologist found 150 cases of negative ulnar variance. 12 of the subjects with negative ulnar variance had Kienböck's disease.

4. Construct the two by two table.

5. Calculate the relative risk for negative ulnar variance as risk factor.

6. Calculate the odds ratio for negative ulnar variance as risk factor.

Chapter 2 - Probability

When flipping a coin, it seems obvious that the chance (or probability) of head is ½ and the chance of tail is also ½. However, what is the probability of two times head in succession? One might think that the probability of this happening is ½ + ½ = 1. However, if the probability is 1 (i.e. 100%), we mean it is a certainty. We all know it is quite possible to have tails three times in succession, so the probability cannot be 1 and should be lower than that.
So, what is the probability of heads twice in succession?

$$½ * ½ = ¼$$

Probabilities are multiplied rather than added.

The example of the coin above is rather unique, in that the probability of heads is equal to the probability of tails (½). Consequently, the probability of heads twice is equal to the probability of tails twice and indeed the probability of heads once and tails once in succession.

So what if we look at a slightly more complicated example; the die?

When rolling a die, the probability of throwing "1" = 1/6. This is equal to the probability of throwing "2", "3", "4", "5" and "6".

As explained above, the probability of twice "1" in succession is:

$$1/6 * 1/6 = 1/36$$

Similarly, the probability of throwing six times "6" is:

$$1/6 * 1/6 * 1/6 * 1/6 * 1/6 * 1/6 = 1/46656 \approx 0.0000214$$

What is the probability of *once* "1", when throwing the die twice?
The probability of this happening is the probability of:

First time "1", second time not "1" : 1/6 * 5/6
First time not "1", second time "1" : 5/6 * 1/6

So the probability is:

1/6 * 5/6 + 5/6 * 1/6 =
5/36 + 5/36 =
10/36 ≈ 0.278 ≈ 28%

So why are these probabilities suddenly added together (rather than multiplied)? The probability of the first time "1" depends on the second time not being "1". These probabilities are therefore dependent and should be multiplied.

Probabilities that are not dependent on each other should be added.

Similarly, we can calculate the probability of the die being *at least once* "1" in two throws. This probability is:

First time "1", second time not "1" : 1/6 * 5/6
First time not "1", second time "1" : 5/6 * 1/6
First time "1" and second time "1" : 1/6 * 1/6

So the probability is:

1/6 * 5/6 + 5/6 * 1/6 + 1/6 * 1/6 =
5/36 + 5/36 + 1/36 =
11/36 ≈ 0.3056 ≈ 31%

Let us look at a slightly more complex example.
What is the probability on twice "1" on throwing a die six times?
One might think this probability would be:

1/6 * 1/6 * 5/6 * 5/6 * 5/6 * 5/6

However, this is the probability of throwing "1" in the first and second throw followed by four throws when the die is not "1". But if we throw a "1" the first and third time we also have thrown "1" twice out of six:

1/6 * 5/6 * 1/6 * 5/6 * 5/6 * 5/6

And if we throw a "1" the first and fourth throw:

1/6 * 5/6 * 5/6 * 1/6 * 5/6 * 5/6

Obviously, there are many combinations possible. If "1" depicts the die being "1" and "x" the die not being "1", the possible combinations are:

```
11xxxx      x11xxx      xx11xx      xxx11x      xxxx11
1x1xxx      x1x1xx      xx1x1x      xxx1x1
1xx1xx      x1xx1x      xx1xx1
1xxx1x      x1xxx1
1xxxx1
```

So there are in total 15 possible combinations. And the probability of throwing "1" twice out of six throws is:

$$1/6 * 1/6 * 5/6 * 5/6 * 5/6 * 5/6 + 1/6 * 5/6 * 1/6 * 5/6 * 5/6 * 5/6 +$$
$$1/6 * 5/6 * 5/6 * 1/6 * 5/6 * 5/6 + .. + 5/6 * 5/6 * 5/6 * 5/6 * 1/6 * 1/6$$

In other words the number of combinations times the probability of one of these combinations:

$$15 * 1/6 * 1/6 * 5/6 * 5/6 * 5/6 * 5/6 \approx 0.201$$

So how do we calculate the number of possible combinations?
The number of possible combinations of two out of six is:

$$\binom{6}{2} \text{ (six over two)}$$

$$\frac{6!}{4!*2!} = \frac{6*5*4*3*2*1}{(4*3*2*1)*(2*1)} = \frac{6*5}{2*1} = \frac{30}{2} = 15$$

In general, the total number of combinations N from n (number of occurrences) out of t (total number of occurrences):

$$N = \binom{t}{n} = \frac{t!}{(t-n)!*(n)!}$$

If c is the probability on a single occurrence; the probability of this not happening is 1-c:

$$\binom{t}{n} * (c)^n * (1-c)^{t-n}$$

So in our example of the die, what is the probability of throwing twice "1" out of six throws?

$$t = 6$$
$$n = 2$$
$$c = 1/6$$

$$\binom{6}{2} * \left(\frac{1}{6}\right)^2 * \left(\frac{5}{6}\right)^{6-2} = \frac{6!}{(6-2)!*(2)!} * \left(\frac{1}{6}\right)^2 * \left(\frac{5}{6}\right)^{6-2} = \frac{6!}{4!*2!} * \left(\frac{1}{6}\right)^2 * \left(\frac{5}{6}\right)^4 =$$

$$\frac{6*5*4*3*2*1}{(4*3*2*1)*(2*1)} * \left(\frac{1}{6}\right)^2 * \left(\frac{5}{6}\right)^4 = \frac{6*5}{2*1} * \left(\frac{1}{6}\right)^2 * \left(\frac{5}{6}\right)^4 = 15 * \frac{1}{6^2} * \frac{5^4}{6^4} =$$

$$15 * \frac{5^4}{6^6} = 15 * \frac{625}{46656} = \frac{9375}{46656} = 0.201$$

What is the probability of throwing *at least* four "6" out of six throws?
This is the probability of throwing 4 times "6" plus the probability of throwing 5 times "6" plus the probability of throwing six times "6":

$$t = 6$$
$$n1 = 4$$
$$n2 = 5$$
$$n3 = 6$$
$$c = 1/6$$

$$\binom{6}{4} * \left(\frac{1}{6}\right)^4 * \left(\frac{5}{6}\right)^{6-4} + \binom{6}{5} * \left(\frac{1}{6}\right)^5 * \left(\frac{5}{6}\right)^{6-5} + \binom{6}{6} * \left(\frac{1}{6}\right)^6 * \left(\frac{5}{6}\right)^{6-6} =$$

$$\frac{6!}{(6-4)!*(4)!} * \left(\frac{1}{6}\right)^4 * \left(\frac{5}{6}\right)^{6-4} + \frac{6!}{(6-5)!*(5)!} * \left(\frac{1}{6}\right)^5 * \left(\frac{5}{6}\right)^{6-5} + 1 * \left(\frac{1}{6}\right)^6 * \left(\frac{5}{6}\right)^0 =$$

$$\frac{6!}{2!*4!} * \left(\frac{1}{6}\right)^4 * \left(\frac{5}{6}\right)^2 + \frac{6!}{1!*5!} * \left(\frac{1}{6}\right)^5 * \left(\frac{5}{6}\right)^1 + 1 * \left(\frac{1}{6}\right)^6 =$$

$$\frac{6*5}{2} * \left(\frac{1}{6}\right)^4 * \left(\frac{5}{6}\right)^2 + \frac{6}{1} * \left(\frac{1}{6}\right)^5 * \left(\frac{5}{6}\right)^1 + 1 * \left(\frac{1}{6}\right)^6 =$$

$$15 * \left(\frac{1^4 * 5^2}{6^6} \right) + 6 * \left(\frac{1^5 * 5^1}{6^6} \right) + 1 * \left(\frac{1^6}{6^6} \right) =$$

$$\frac{15 * 5^2 + 6 * 5 + 1}{6^6} \approx 0.0087 \approx 1\%$$

Please note that $\binom{6}{4} = \binom{6}{2} = 15$ and that $\binom{6}{6} = \binom{6}{0} = 1$

In general, $\binom{t}{n} = \binom{t}{t-n}$.

So far, we have only been concerned with probabilities that do **not** change. Our examples of the coin and die are similar to putting ten balls (numbered 1 to 10) in a hat; taking one out and **putting it back** afterwards. In that case, the probability of getting ball number "1" once is 1/10 and getting it twice in succession is 1/10 * 1/10 = 1/100. The probability of getting ball number "1" twice out of four draws is:

$$\binom{t}{n} * (c)^n * (1-c)^{t-n}$$

c = 1/10
t = 4
n = 2

$$\binom{4}{2} * \left(\frac{1}{10} \right)^2 * \left(\frac{9}{10} \right)^2 =$$

$$\frac{4!}{2! * 2!} * \left(\frac{1}{10} \right)^2 * \left(\frac{9}{10} \right)^2 =$$

$$\frac{4 * 3}{2 * 1} * \left(\frac{1}{10} \right)^2 * \left(\frac{9}{10} \right)^2 =$$

$$6 * \left(\frac{1 * 9^2}{10^4} \right) = 0.0486 \approx 5\%$$

However, often we have to deal with situations were the probability depends on the previous history. In other words, taking the balls out of the hat **without putting them back**!

If we start with all ten balls in the hat, the probability of drawing number "1" is 1/10. The probability on a successive ball ("2", "3", "4", "5", "6", "7", "8", "9" 0r "10") is now 1/9.

The probability that we draw number "1" followed by number "5" is 1/10 * 1/9. This is equal to the probability we draw number "5" followed by number "1".

So in drawing two balls, the probability we draw ball number "1" and ball number "5" in any order is:

2 * 1/10 *1 /9 ≈ 0.022 ≈ 2%

So how do we calculate the probability in more complicated scenarios? It has to be remembered that the probability on X happening equals the number of possible combinations with X divided by the total number of possible combinations:

$$\textbf{Probability (X)} = \frac{\text{Number of Combinations with X}}{\text{Total Number of Combinations}}$$

So how do we calculate the possible number of combinations? We have already seen that the number of combinations N equals:

$$N = \binom{t}{n} = \frac{t!}{(t-n)!*(n)!}$$

The number of combinations of getting one ball out of the hat is obviously:

$$\binom{1}{1} = 1$$

So the probability of getting the ball with number "1" out of the hat with ten balls is:

$$\frac{\binom{1}{1}}{\binom{10}{1}} = \frac{1}{\frac{10!}{9!*1!}} = \frac{9!}{10!} = \frac{1}{10}$$

Which is what we calculated previously.

Similarly, getting number "1" and number "5" in any order is:

$$\frac{\binom{1}{1}*\binom{1}{1}}{\binom{10}{2}} = \frac{1}{\frac{10!}{8!*2!}} = \frac{8!*2!}{10!} = \frac{2}{10*9} \approx 0.022 \approx 2\%$$

The number of combinations in the numerator should be multiplied, as they depend on each other.

In more general terms:

$$\text{Probability (X)} = \frac{\binom{z}{a}*\binom{x}{b}*\binom{y}{c}}{\binom{t}{n}}$$

t = total number of occurrences
n = number of occurrences
t = *z* + *x* + *y*
n = *a* + *b* + *c*

So let us look at playing cards.
What is the probability on getting one king when we draw five cards?

There are four kings in the set, so there are

$$\binom{4}{1}$$ Possibilities

The remaining four cards should not be kings. There are 51 cards left, of which three are kings and 48 non kings. So the number of possibilities on selecting four cards that are not kings is:

$$\binom{48}{4}$$

The total number of possibilities on selecting five cards out of 52 is obviously:

$$\binom{52}{5}$$

So the probability of getting one King is:

$$\frac{\binom{4}{1}*\binom{48}{4}}{\binom{52}{5}} = \frac{\frac{4!}{3!*1!}*\frac{48!}{44!*4!}}{\frac{52!}{47!*5!}} = \frac{4!*48!*47!*5!}{3!*1!*44!*4!*52!} = \frac{48!*47!*5!}{3!*44!*52!} =$$

$$\frac{48!*47!*5!}{52!*44!*3!} = \frac{47*46*45*5*4}{52*51*50*49} = \frac{1945800}{6497400} \approx 0.299 \approx 30\%$$

It should be noted that 4 + 48 = 52 and 1 + 4 = 5.

Let us calculate the probability of drawing any one king, the queen of hearts and a further queen out of a total five playing cards.
We start with the number of possibilities of drawing one king:

$$\binom{4}{1}$$

Now the Queen of hearts:

$$\binom{1}{1}$$

There are three queens remaining, so the number of possibilities on drawing one further queen is:

$$\binom{3}{1}$$

Followed by two cards that are neither a king nor a remaining queen (there are in total 44 non kings and queens in the set).

$$\binom{44}{2}$$

It should be noted that 4 + 1 + 3 + 44 = 52 and 1 + 1 + 1 + 2 = 5.

The total number of possible combinations is as previously:

$$\binom{52}{5}$$

So the probability of drawing any one king, the queen of hearts and a further queen out of a total five playing cards is:

$$\frac{\binom{4}{1}*\binom{1}{1}*\binom{3}{1}*\binom{44}{2}}{\binom{52}{5}} = \frac{\dfrac{4!}{3!*1!}*1*\dfrac{3!}{2!*1!}*\dfrac{44!}{42!*2!}}{\dfrac{52!}{47!*5!}} = \frac{4!*3!*44!*47!*5!}{3!*2!*42!*2!*52!} =$$

$$\frac{47!*44!*5!*4!*3!}{52!*42!*3!*2!*2!} = \frac{44*43*5*4*3*4*3}{52*51*50*49*48} = \frac{1362240}{311875200} \approx$$

0.0044 ≈ 0.4%

Summary Chapter 2

- **Probabilities that are dependent are multiplied**

- **Probabilities that are not dependent are added**

- Probability (X) = $\dfrac{\text{Number of Combinations with X}}{\text{Total Number of Combinations}}$

- Number of combinations N:

  $$N = \binom{t}{n} = \frac{t!}{(t-n)! * (n)!}$$

  t = total number of occurrences

  n = number of occurrences

- Probability (X) = $\binom{t}{n} * (c)^n * (1-c)^{t-n}$ (with putting back)

  t = total number of occurrences

  n = number of occurrences

  c = probability on single occurrence

- Probability (X) = $\dfrac{\binom{z}{a} * \binom{x}{b} * \binom{y}{c}}{\binom{t}{n}}$ (without putting back)

  t = total number of occurrences

  n = number of occurrences

  $t = z + x + y$

  $n = a + b + c$

Questions Chapter 2

1. When rolling a ten sided die, calculate the probability on three times "7" out of ten throws.

2. There are 20 different objects. Of these 9 should be painted red, 8 white and 3 blue. How many combinations are there?

3. What is the probability of drawing 1 king, the queen of hearts and two further queens out of a normal deck of playing cards when five cards are drawn?

4. What is the probability of drawing 1 king, the queen of hearts and no further queens out of a normal deck of playing cards when five cards are drawn?

5. What is the probability of drawing *at least* one king out of normal deck of playing cards when five cards are drawn?

6. What is the probability of winning the lottery, when you need to have all six numbers from a total of 49 correct?

Chapter 3 – Data & Distribution of Data

Data Types

Data is something we measure. This could for example be height, function or quality of life. Data can be qualitative or quantitative.

Qualitative data arise when people fall into *different classes*. There are two different types of qualitative data: nominal and ordinal.

> ***Nominal data***
>> The data consists of different classes that can ***not be ranked***. For example groups of patients who had a *wedge osteotomy* compared to patients who had a *dome osteotomy*.

> ***Ordinal data***
>> The data can be ***ranked***.
>> For example outcome of patients is classed as *walking with a frame*, *walking with a stick* and *walking unaided*. So, there is an order in the data.

Quantitative data are numerical. They can be either whole numbers (integer) or any number (real numbers).
If the data are integer, they are called ***discrete***. Data that can be any real number is called ***continuous data***.

Let us assume we have a group of 100 people and we want to measure their height (continuous data).
The height is called the ***variable*** we measure:

Variable: Actual property measured by individual observations

Every person in the group will have an individual height measurement. This individual measurement is called the ***variate***:

Variate: Single score or reading of a given variable

Normal Distribution

We have measured the height of 100 people to the nearest centimetre. So, the measured variable is height and there are 100 variates. There were 5 people with a height of 168 cm, 25 with a height of 169 cm, 40 with a height of 170 cm, 25 with a height of 171 cm and 5 with a height of 172 cm. The results are shown in the table below.

Height	Number
168	5
169	25
170	40
171	25
172	5
Total	**100**

We can also plot the data in a graph:

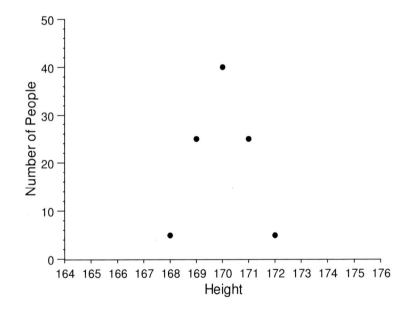

If we connect the data points, we get the distribution graph:

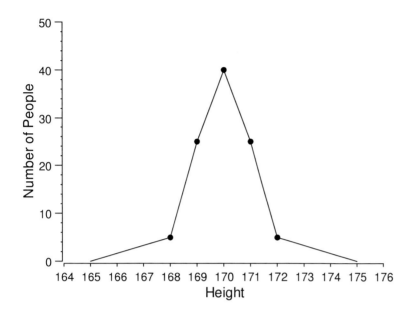

If we would measure in millimetres rather than centimetres (greater precision; see chapter 7) and fit a smooth curve through the data, we get the distribution graph:

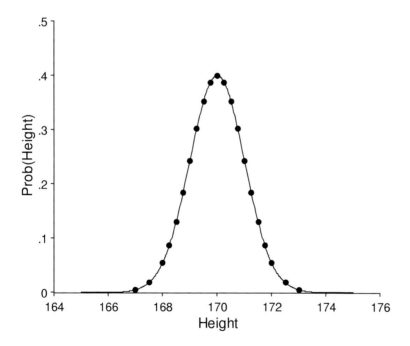

This graph shows the **distribution** of the variable height.

Also note that the y-axis now shows the **probability** rather than the actual number of people.

This curve is called the **Gaussian or 'bell shaped' curve**.

The curve has the following basic formula:

$$y = \frac{1}{\sqrt{2\pi}} \exp\left(-\frac{x^2}{2}\right)$$

Further mathematics is beyond the scope of this book.
However, if data are distributed according to this formula, the data are called **normally distributed**.
Any other distribution of data is called a **non normal**.
This has important implications for statistical tests that can be used (chapter 5). Only if the data is normally distributed can parametric statistics be used. If this is not the case, non parametric statistics should be used (chapter 5).

Mean

If we return to the example above, we can calculate the mean height.
The mean height is:

$$\text{Mean height} = \frac{5*168 + 25*169 + 40*170 + 25*171 + 5*172}{100} = 170 \text{ cm}$$

As can be seen, the mean is at the top of the Gaussian curve.
The curve is symmetrical around the mean.

Or in general the mean is:

$$\bar{x} = \frac{1}{n} \sum_{i=1}^{n} x_i$$

The mean and average are often used as synonyms. However, they are *not* quite the same.
The mean is an average, but there are *other* averages apart from the mean (such as mode and median). They will be discussed later in this chapter (non normal distributions).

Let us look at a distribution with mean zero and standard deviation of 1:

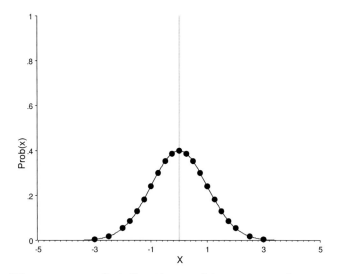

The same distribution with mean -1:

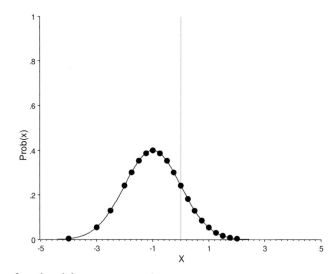

And with mean +1:

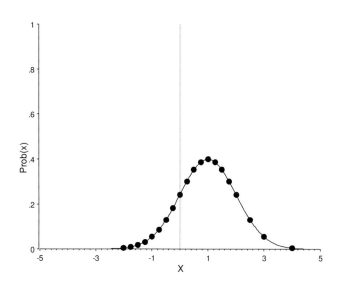

As can be seen; the distribution curve shifts to the left when the mean decreases and to the right when the mean increases. The shape of the curve however, remains unchanged:

A different mean shifts the curve along the x-axis, but does not alter its shape.

Standard Deviation & Variance

In describing normally distributed data, the standard deviation and variance are used. They are a measure of the **spread (or variability)** of the data. The variance is the standard deviation (S) squared or:

$$Variance = (S)^2$$

Or:

$$S = \sqrt{Variance}$$

The variance is defined as follows:

$$Variance = \frac{1}{n-1}\sum (x_i - \overline{x})^2 \qquad (\overline{x} \text{ is the mean})$$

The term $\sum (x_i - \overline{x})^2$ is the *sum of the squares about the mean*.

If we return to our example:

Height	Number
168	5
169	25
170	40
171	25
172	5
Total	**100**

As calculated above, the mean is 170.

The sum of the squares about the mean is:

$$\sum\left(x_i - \overline{x}\right)^2 =$$

$$= 5*(168 - 170)^2 + 25*(169 - 170)^2 + 40*(170 - 170)^2 +$$

$$25*(171 - 170)^2 + 5*(172 - 170)^2 =$$

$$= 5*(-2)^2 + 25*(-1)^2 + 40*(0)^2 + 25*(1)^2 + 5*(2)^2 =$$

$$= 5*4 + 25*1 + 40*0 + 25*1 + 5*4$$

$$= 20 + 25 + 25 + 20 = 90$$

So the variance is:

$$Variance = \frac{1}{100 - 1} * 90 \approx 0.91$$

And the standard deviation is:

$$S = \sqrt{0.91} \approx 0.95$$

Again, let us look at a normal distribution with a mean of zero and a standard deviation of 1:

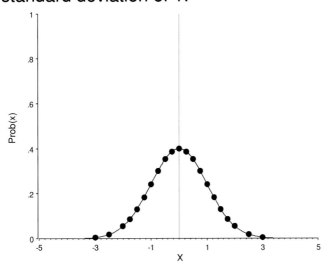

The same distribution, but with standard deviation 0.5:

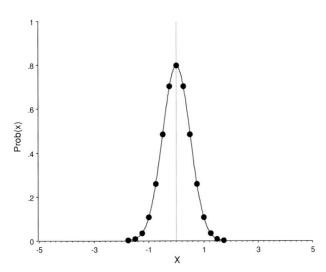

And with standard deviation 2:

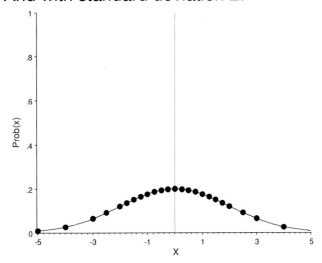

So the standard deviation is a measure of the spread (or variability of the data).

When the standard deviation decreases, the curve becomes steeper (data closer together).

When the standard deviation increases, the curve becomes flatter (data further spread apart).

If the data are normally distributed, the distribution of data can be described by two parameters: the mean and the standard deviation (or variance).

As stated above, the standard deviation is a measure of the spread of data. It can be shown that 68.27% of the data lie in an interval plus or minus one standard deviation from the mean. Similarly 95.45% of the data lie in an interval plus or minus twice the standard deviation and 99.73% of the data within an interval plus or minus three times the standard deviation.
Or:

Mean + / - 1 * SD = 68 %
Mean + / - 2 * SD = 95 %
Mean + / - 3 * SD = 99 %

This is shown in graphs on the next page.

Mean + or – 1 times standard deviation (68% of the data in interval):

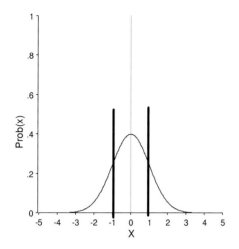

Mean + or – 2 times standard deviation (95% of the data in interval):

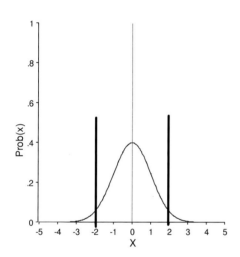

Mean + or - 3 times standard deviation (99% of the data in interval):

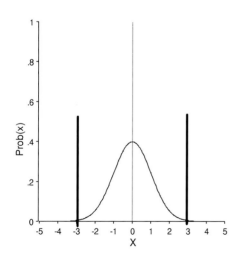

In our previous example, the Mean was 170 and the standard deviation was 0.95.
So:

> 68% of the data are between 169.05 and 170.95
> 95% of the data are between 168.1 and 171.9
> 99% of the data are between 167.15 and 172.85

Non Normal Distributions

The normal distribution is the most widely studied distribution amongst statitcians. As stated above, the curve is 'bell shaped' and has a general formula of:

$$y = \frac{1}{\sqrt{2\pi}} \exp\left(-\frac{x^2}{2}\right)$$

The distribution can only be called normal if it follows this general formula. Any other distribution is called non normal.
There are many types of distributions and it is impossible to name them all. Common examples are curves that are skewed either to the left or right.

As stated above, normal distributions can be described with a mean and standard deviation (or variance).
Non normal distributions require many more parameters to describe them.

It is common to use the range:

Range: Interval from lowest to highest value

As in a normal distribution, we can calculate a mean (average) with:

$$\bar{x} = \frac{1}{n} \sum_{i=1}^{n} x_i$$

As can be seen in the example below, the curve is **not** necessarily symmetrical around the mean:

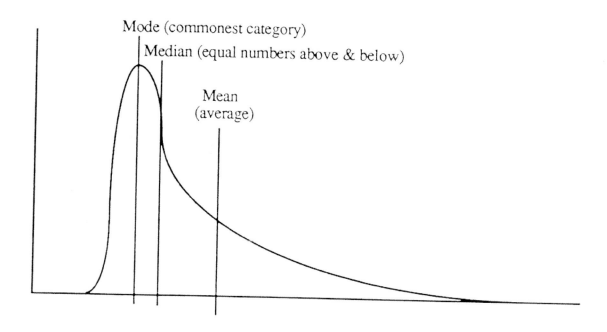

Other averages that are used to describe non normal distributions are the mode and median.

Mode: **Most common category**

Median: **Equal number of measurements above and below**

(In the normal distribution: the mode, median and mean are the same!)

It is of course possible to calculate a standard deviation in non normal distributed data. However, hopefully it is obvious from the graph above that this makes no sense. Certainly in that case, it can **not** be said that 68% of the data lie in an interval between plus or minus one standard deviation from the mean!

Summary Chapter 3

Qualitative data	**Different classes**
Nominal	**Not ranked**
Ordinal	**Ranked**
Quantitative data	**Numerical**
Discrete	**Integer number**
Continuous	**Real number**

Variable: Actual property measured by individual observations

Variate: Single score or reading of a given variable

Normal distribution:

$$y = \frac{1}{\sqrt{2\pi}} \exp\left(\frac{x^2}{2}\right)$$

Mean:

$$\bar{x} = \frac{1}{n}\sum_{i=1}^{n} x_i$$

A different mean shifts the curve along the x-axis, but does not alter its shape.

$$Variance = \frac{1}{n-1}\sum\left(x_i - \bar{x}\right)^2$$

$$S = \sqrt{Variance}$$

(S = standard deviation)

When the standard deviation decreases, the curve becomes steeper; when the standard deviation increases, the curve becomes flatter.

If the data is normally distributed, the distribution of data can be described by two parameters:
- **Mean**
- **Standard deviation   (or variance)**

Mean + / - 1 * SD = 68 %
Mean + / - 2 * SD = 95 %
Mean + / - 3 * SD = 99 %

Non normal distribution:

Range: Interval from lowest to highest value

Mode: Most common category

Median: Equal number of measurements above and below

Chapter 4 – Growth Curves, Z-Scores & T-Scores

Growth curves, Percentiles and Quantiles

Below are typical growth curves for boys:

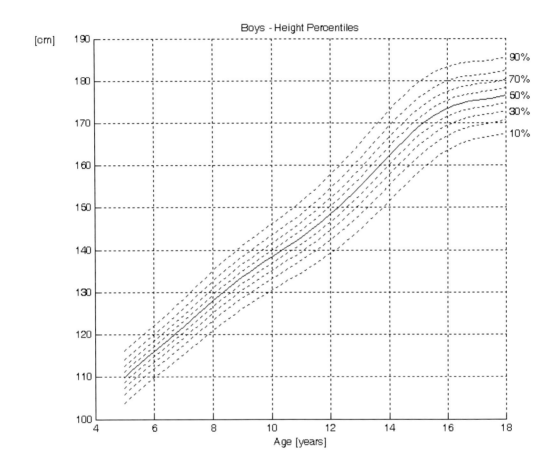

And girls:

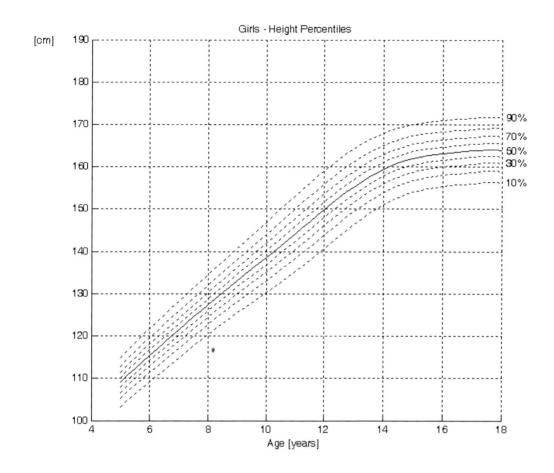

The curves show the height as function of the age for boys and girls.

The dotted lines are the percentiles. They indicate the proportion of children that are below a certain height. Ten per cent of the children are below the 10th percentile in height and consequently 90% are above it. Similarly, 30 per cent of the children are below the 30th percentile and 70 per cent above it. Also, 70 per cent are below the 70th percentile and 30 per cent above it.

The 50th percentile is shown as a solid line.
Indeed, 50 per cent of the children are taller than the 50th percentile and 50 per cent shorter.
It can be demonstrated that height is normally distributed (chapter 3). Therefore, in growth curves, the 50th percentile (P50) is the same as the mean (average) and the mode and the median.

P50 = mean = mode = median

It can be read from the growth curves above, that the mean final height for boys is approximately 176 cm, whilst this is 164 cm for girls.
Twelve year old girls are on average 150 cm tall, whilst boys this age are approximately 148 cm.

From these curves, it can be seen that girls reach skeletal maturity earlier than boys. The curve for girls reaches a plateau at 15 years of age, whilst this is approximately 17 years for boys.

Quantiles are similar to percentiles.
As the name implies, quantiles divide the data in four groups. The first quantile is at 25%, the second at 50%, the third at 75% and the fourth at 100%. So, the 25th percentile is the same as the first quantile.
The 2nd quantile line is the same as the 50th percentile, the median, mode and median.

P50 = mean = mode = median = 2nd quantile

Growth curves with quantiles are shown on the next page. Only the 1st, 2nd and 3rd quantiles are shown:

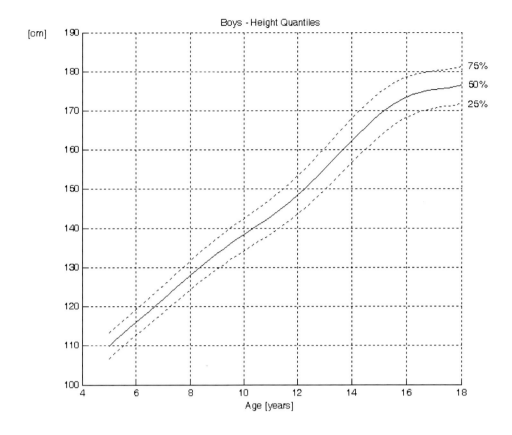

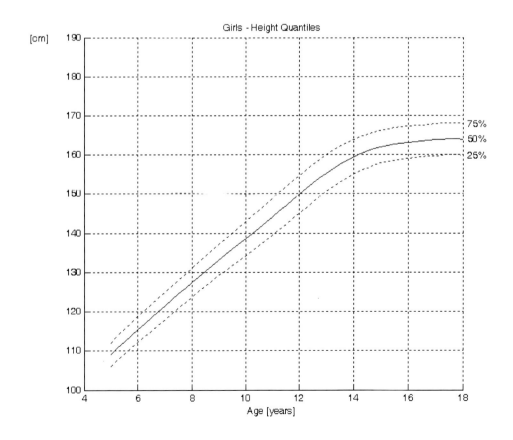

As stated previously, height is normally distributed. At any particular age, the percentiles show a Gaussian or bell shaped curve. The growth charts are a **continuum of Gaussian curves**. This is shown three dimensionally below:

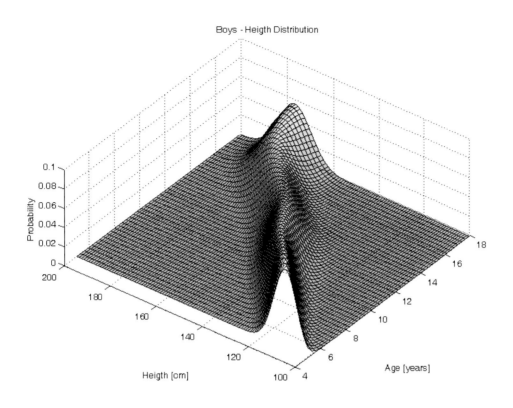

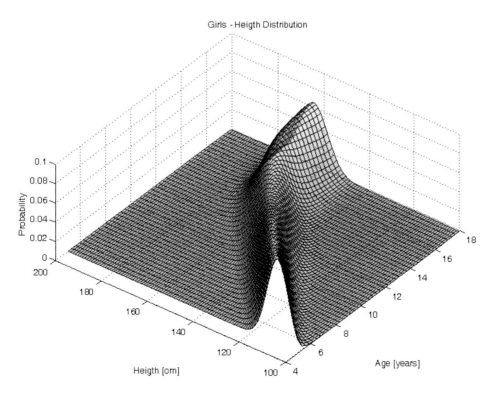

It was shown in chapter 3 that, in normally distributed data, 68.27% of the data lie in an interval plus or minus one standard deviation from the mean. Similarly 95.45% of the data lie in an interval plus or minus twice the standard deviation and 99.73% of the data within an interval plus or minus three times the standard deviation.

Or:
Mean + / - 1 * SD = 68.27 %
Mean + / - 2 * SD = 95.45 %
Mean + / - 3 * SD = 99.73 %

To 'translate' this into percentiles:

One standard deviation about the mean:
68.27 % about the mean (P50) is the interval between

$50 - (68.27 / 2) = 50 - 34.135 = 15.865 \approx 16^{th}$ percentile
and
$50 + (68.27 / 2) = 50 + 34.135 = 84.135 \approx 84^{th}$ percentile

Similarly, two standard deviations about the mean:

$50 - (95.45 / 2) = 50 - 47.725 = 2.275 \approx 2^{nd}$ percentile
and
$50 + (95.45 / 2) = 50 + 47.725 = 97.725 \approx 98^{th}$ percentile

And three:

$50 - (99.73 / 2) = 50 - 49.865 = 0.135 \approx 0.1^{th}$ percentile
and
$50 + (99.73 / 2) = 50 + 49.865 = 99.865 \approx 99.9^{th}$ percentile

In summary:

Mean + / - 1 * SD = 68.27 % : between 16th and 84th percentile
Mean + / - 2 * SD = 95.45 % : between 2nd and 98th percentile
Mean + / - 3 * SD = 99.73 % : between 0.1^{th} and 99.9^{th} percentile

Z-Scores

Obviously, the mean height is different for children of different age. Children are growing and their height increases with age.
It is important to know whether a child grows sufficiently as compared to its peers. Therefore, standardisation is required. Z-scores were introduced for this purpose. The child's height is expressed as how many standard deviations it is above or below the mean.

Z-score = (height – mean height) / standard deviation

The growth charts show that the average height for a twelve year old girl is 150 cm.
A child of average height has a z-score of 0:
(150-150) / standard deviation = 0 / standard deviation = 0

What about twelve year old girl who is 160 cm?
The z-score is:
(160-150) / standard deviation
The standard deviation can be estimated from the growth chart.
It was shown above that the mean + / - one standard deviation is between the 16th and 84th percentile.
The 16th percentile for a twelve year old girl is approximately 142 cm (read from chart). Therefore, the standard deviation is 150 – 142 = 8 cm.
So, the z-score is (160-150) / 8 = 10 / 8 = 1.25
She is one and a quarter standard deviations above the mean for her age.

Similarly, a twelve year old girl who is 125 cm has a z-score of:
Z-score = (125 – 150) / 8 = (-25) / 8 = -3.125. She is more than 3 standard deviations below the average for her age.

Z-scores are very useful in follow up of children and comparing their growth rate with their peers.
Assume a five year old child has a z-score of -1 (one standard deviation below the average height for a five year old).
If the child has a z-score of -2 when 10 years old, the rate of growth has been less than its peers and this could indicate malnutrition or disease.
If the child has a z-score of 0 when 10 years old, the rate of growth has exceeded that of its peers.
Finally, if the child has a z-score of -1 when 10 years old, the rate of growth has been the same as its peers. The child however remains smaller than average and one standard deviation below the mean.

In summary, a change is z-score indicates a difference in growth rate as compared to the normal population. An increase in z-score indicates a growth rate greater than average and a decrease in z-score a growth rate less than average. If the z-score remains the same, the rate of growth is the same as the normal population.

T-Scores

Z-scores can also be used to express bone mineral density.
The bone mineral density is referenced to the mean for that age:

A z-score is the number of standard deviations the bone mineral density measurement is above or below the *age-matched mean* bone mineral density.

Z-score = (BMD – *age-matched mean* BMD) / standard deviation
(BMD = bone mineral density)

However, to define osteoporosis the bone mineral density in a young normal is used as reference. This is the t-score:

A t-score is the number of standard deviations the bone mineral density measurement is above or below the *young-normal mean* bone mineral density.

T-score = (BMD – *young-normal mean* BMD) / standard deviation
(BMD = bone mineral density)

The World Health Organisation defined osteoporosis / osteopenia in 1994. Four diagnostic categories were defined based on bone mineral density. The t-score, using young adult women as the referent group, defines the diagnostic categories:

- Normal: t-score -1 or above

- Osteopenia: t-score between -1 and -2.5

- Osteoporosis: t-score less than -2.5

- Severe osteoporosis: t-score less than -2.5 and fragility fracture

The graph below shows the forearm bone mineral density as function of the age:

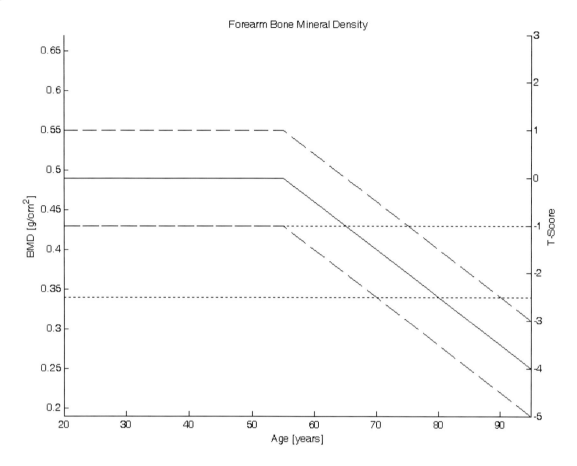

The left hand y-axis indicates the bone mineral density in gram per centimetre square. The corresponding t-score is based on the bone mineral density in a 20 year old and shown on the right hand y-axis.

The solid line indicates the mean bone mineral density and the dashed lines one standard deviation away from the mean. Therefore, 68% of the people have a bone mineral density between the two dashed lines (above and chapter 3).

The two horizontal dotted lines show the osteopenia limit (t-score = -1) and the osteoporosis limit (t-score = -2.5).

Z-scores are less commonly used than t-scores, but may be helpful in identifying persons who should undergo a work-up for secondary causes of osteoporosis. Z-scores and t-scores can be converted into each other using a reference table provided the age, gender, race and skeletal site are known.

Neither the z-score not the t-score can predict fracture risk on its own. It is also necessary to know the age of the patient. Because t-scores and z-scores can be converted into each other, fracture risk can be predicted with either.

Consider the patient in the graph below:

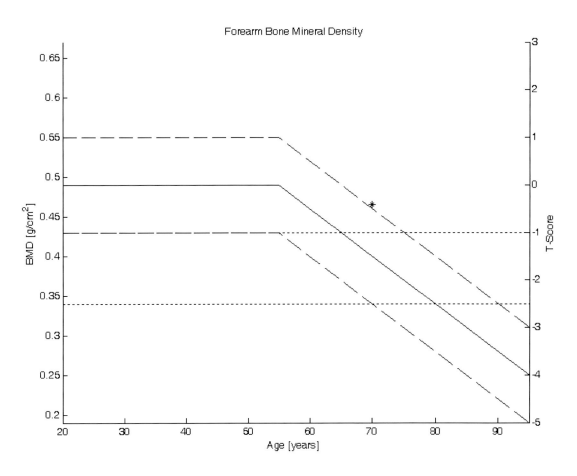

Patient

Age:	70 years
Bone mineral density:	0.465 g/cm^2
Z-score:	**+1**

Young normal (20 years)

Mean bone density:	0.49 g/cm^2
Standard deviation bone density:	0.49 – 0.43 = 0.06 g/cm^2
T-score:	(0.465 – 0.49) / 0.06 = -0.025 / 0.06 = **-0.42**
WHO category:	**Normal**

Also, the bone density measurement of the 90 years old lady with a fracture neck of femur:

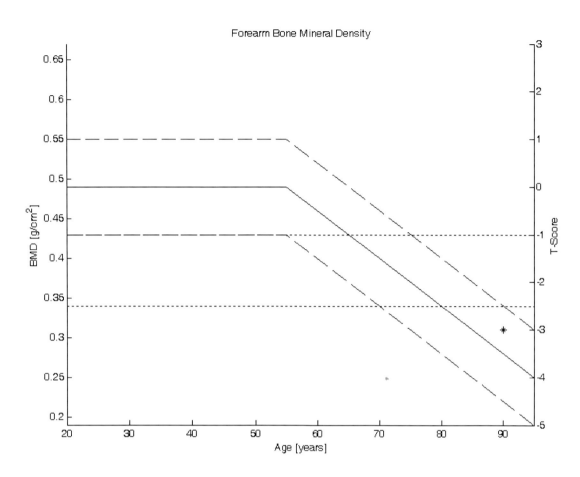

Patient

Age:	90 years
Bone mineral density:	0.31 g/cm^2
Z-score:	**≈ +0.5**

Young normal (20 years)

Mean bone density:	0.49 g/cm^2
Standard deviation bone density:	0.49 – 0.43 = 0.06 g/cm^2
T-score:	(0.31 – 0.49) / 0.06 = -0.18 / 0.06 = **-3**
WHO category:	**Severe osteoporosis**

Summary Chapter 4

- **Growth curves:**
  P50 = mean = mode = median = 2nd quantile

- **Mean $+/- 1 * SD = 68.27$ % :**
  between 16th and 84th percentile
  Mean $+/- 2 * SD = 95.45$ % :
  between 2nd and 98th percentile
  Mean $+/- 3 * SD = 99.73$ % :
  between 0.1^{th} and 99.9^{th} percentile

- **Z-score = (height − mean height) / standard deviation**

- **A z-score is the number of standard deviations the bone mineral density measurement is above or below the *age-matched mean* bone mineral density**

- **Z-score =**
  (BMD − *age-matched mean* BMD) / standard deviation
  (BMD = bone mineral density)

- **A t-score is the number of standard deviations the bone mineral density measurement is above or below the *young-normal mean* bone mineral density**

- **T-score =**
  (BMD − *young-normal mean* BMD) / standard deviation
  (BMD = bone mineral density)

- **World Health Organisation definition (1994):**

  Normal: t-score -1 or above

  Osteopenia: t-score between -1 and -2.5

  Osteoporosis: t-score less than -2.5

  Severe osteoporosis: t-score less than -2.5 and

                         fragility fracture

Chapter 5 – Statistical Tests

Hypothesis

We are interested in finding out if there is a difference in nutritional status in patients who present to our outpatient department with cancer as compared to patients who do not have cancer.
Our impression is that patients with cancer have a nutritional status that is worse than other patients. We would like to test if this impression is correct.

In order to test this statement, we need to formulate a **hypothesis**.
The null hypothesis states that there is no difference between the two groups of patients.

Null hypothesis: **No difference between study groups**

As an alternative there is the alternate hypothesis:

Alternate hypothesis: **There is a difference between groups (worse *or* better nutrition)**

It does seem perhaps a bit strange, but it is common practice in statistical testing to formulate a null hypothesis (ie there is no difference) and then try to refute this hypothesis with a statistical test.

With our statistical test we are trying to prove if the null hypothesis is incorrect.

First, we need to define an **outcome measure**. We could use several variables for this (such as albumin concentration in peripheral blood, body mass index etc). We decided to use the thickness of the biceps skin fold as our outcome measure.
So, the variable we use as our outcome measure is the biceps skin fold thickness. We measure this with a special instrument that measures the thickness of the skin fold in millimetres. The data collected is therefore continuous data (chapter 3).

Next, we need to know how certain we would like to be.
In first instance one would say 100%! However, nothing is certain (and not even that!).

P Value & Significance

Statistics deals with uncertainty. When we make a statement; we also need to say how certain we are that this statement is correct. We would like this to be 100%, but realise that this is not possible.

It is generally accepted (in medical statistics) that something is 'proven' if we are more than 95% certain. This means that there is a probability of 5% that our statement is *incorrect*. Or ***p = 5%.***

P Value   Probability that statement is incorrect

We usually call something 'proven' or ***statistically significant*** if following a statistical test the p value < 5%.

Statistically significant   p < 5%

That something is statistically significant doesn't necessarily mean it is also ***clinically significant***. It might well be that, although statistically there is a difference, it is of no clinical importance.

Also, if we were unable to demonstrate a statistically significant difference; this doesn't mean there is no difference. After all, if p = 5% there is a probability of 1 in 20 that our statement is incorrect! It might well be that with more patients in our study, we can demonstrate a significant difference.

If p = 5%, there is a probability of 1 in 20 that our statement is incorrect. However, in 19 out of 20 times our statement is correct.

In a lot of cases we would like to be more certain than this (when we cross the road or fly in a plane!). Also when we buy a bottle of wine, we wouldn't accept it if one in 20 bottles has less than 75 cl of wine!

If p = 1%, our statement is incorrect only 1 out of 100; whilst this is 1 in 1000 if p = 0.1%. The *smaller* the p value the *more* certain we are that what we say is true. Consequently, we aim for a *low* p value.

However, the lower the p value, the more patients would be required to demonstrate a statistically significant difference. Furthermore, in biological systems (unlike man made systems) the variation is large. Therefore, it is very unlikely to get p values much below 5% or 1%. If the p value is considerably lower than 1% it is more likely that we are trying to state the obvious or that the variables are dependent.

In medical statistics we are usually satisfied something is statistically significant if p < 5%. If p < 5%, we feel this is unlikely to be due to chance and the null hypothesis is rejected in favour of the alternate hypothesis.

Let us return to our example.

The next 29 patients that attended our outpatient department had their biceps skin fold measured. The results are shown in the table below. The data are *not* in order of when the patient attended outpatient clinic, but grouped by diagnosis and increasing thickness of the skin fold. Patients either had 'No Cancer' or 'Cancer':

1	No Cancer	1.9
2	No Cancer	2.2
3	No Cancer	2.3
4	No Cancer	2.6
5	No Cancer	2.8
6	No Cancer	2.9
7	No Cancer	3
8	No Cancer	3.7
9	No Cancer	3.8
10	No Cancer	4
11	No Cancer	4.3
12	No Cancer	4.4
13	No Cancer	4.8
14	No Cancer	5.6
15	No Cancer	6
16	No Cancer	6.2
17	No Cancer	6.2
18	No Cancer	7
19	No Cancer	10
20	No Cancer	10.4
21	Cancer	1.8
22	Cancer	2
23	Cancer	2
24	Cancer	2
25	Cancer	3
26	Cancer	3.8
27	Cancer	3.9
28	Cancer	4
29	Cancer	4.1

We call the difference significant if p < 5%.

Now we need to decide which **statistical test** to use.

A statistical test can either be **parametric** or **non parametric**.

A parametric test can **only** be used if the data are **normally distributed** (chapter 3). If the data are not normally distributed, we can **not** use parametric statistics and we will have to use a non parametric test. We will discuss parametric tests first, followed by non parametric tests.

Parametric Tests

As stated above, parametric tests can **only** be used if the data are normally distributed. Therefore, the data need to be continuous data. However, continuous data are not necessarily normally distributed, and the data could well be skewed.

Often, we do not know how data are distributed and it is difficult to tell from our sample what the distribution of data is. The distribution could be normal; but we are not sure. It this case we can use a statistical test to test whether the data is normally distributed or not. There are several test described to **test for normality**. An example is the Shapiro-Wilk test. However, a description of these tests is beyond the scope of this book.

If we have a **large sample size** (>50) we can use the normal distribution itself and read from the graph. Usually, we perform a **two sided** test. This means that the alternate hypothesis could be bigger **or** smaller than the null hypothesis. Consequently, we have to 'share' the 5% between the two tail ends of the curve (2.5% at each tail end):

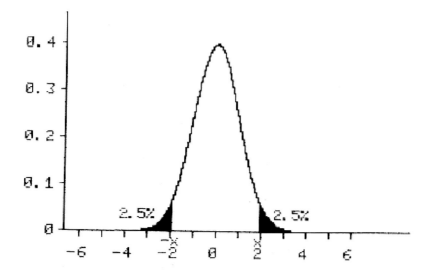

It should be noted that this is plus or minus twice the standard deviation from the mean (chapter 3).
So, if the mean of our study group lies in each of the two dark areas on the graph; we feel this is very unlikely to be due to chance and the null hypothesis is rejected in favour of the alternate hypothesis.

Occasionally, we know that the alternate hypothesis can only be larger than the alternate hypothesis. In that case we can use the 5% on only one tail end of the curve. This is called **one sided** testing.

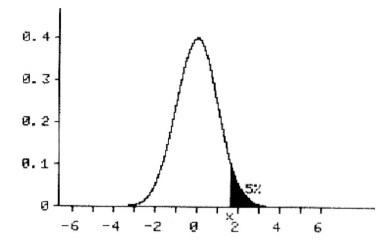

t-Test

As stated above, if the sample size is large (> 50), we can use the normal distribution and read from the graph. However, it is only rarely we have such large sample size. Usually our sample sizes are much smaller (around 20 to 30). In this case we can not use the normal distribution and have to correct for the small sample size. This can be done using the **t-test**.

In our example, let us assume we have demonstrated that the data are normally distributed (with a test for normality). We can now use the t-test to analyse the data. A mathematical description of the t-test is beyond the scope of this book. Suffice to say that the t-test corrects for the smaller sample size with a 'correction factor'.
If we feed our data in a computer we can perform an **unpaired t-test**. We group by 'disease' ('No Cancer' or 'Cancer'). The **grouping variable** is the column 'disease' (nominal data):

Group Info for Skin Fold
Grouping Variable: Disease

	Count	Mean	Variance	Std. Dev.	Std. Err
Cancer	9	2.956	1.010	1.005	.335
No Cancer	20	4.705	5.759	2.400	.537

57

The computer calculates the p Value using the t-test:

Unpaired t-test for Skin Fold
Grouping Variable: Disease
Hypothesized Difference = 0

	Mean Diff.	DF	t-Value	P-Value
Cancer, No Cancer	-1.749	27	-2.089	.0462

P = 4.62% < 5%
Therefore, the probability that the difference is due to chance is very small and the difference is statistically significant. We can therefore reject the null hypothesis in favour of the alternate hypothesis. So we conclude that there is a difference in skin fold thickness in patients with cancer and that their nutrition is poorer.

In the example above, the t-test was performed on one sample of data. We can also perform a t-test on two samples.
If the data are dependent, we use a ***paired t-test***. Otherwise, we use an **unpaired t-test**.
An example of dependent data is the range of movement in the knee before and after a total knee replacement. We have two groups of data: range of movement before and after total knee replacement. The two groups are dependent and provided the data in normally distributed; we can use the paired t-test.
We can use a paired t-test before and after a process of change, or in the same subject measured at different times.

Non Parametric Tests

If data are not normally distributed, we have to use a non parametric test. There are many non parametric tests described, and it is impossible to name / lists them all. We will discuss three tests; using our skin fold example:

- **Sign test**
- **Chi Square test**
- **Mann Whitney U test**

In the example with the skin fold measurement, we used the t-test. From now on, let us assume the data is not normally distributed. Therefore, we can not use parametric statistics and will have to use non parametric statistics. We analyse the data with each of the three tests above.

Sign Test

This is the most basic type of non parametric test. As the name implies, it uses the plus or minus sign to differentiate. The reader might want to return to chapter 2 to remind him or her self about the calculation of probabilities. First we transform the data. If the skin fold is smaller or equal to 4 mm, we indicate this by a minus and if the skin fold is greater than 4 mm by a plus sign.

Returning to our data table:

1	No Cancer	1.9	-
2	No Cancer	2.2	-
3	No Cancer	2.3	-
4	No Cancer	2.6	-
5	No Cancer	2.8	-
6	No Cancer	2.9	-
7	No Cancer	3	-
8	No Cancer	3.7	-
9	No Cancer	3.8	-
10	No Cancer	4	-
11	No Cancer	4.3	+
12	No Cancer	4.4	+
13	No Cancer	4.8	+
14	No Cancer	5.6	+
15	No Cancer	6	+
16	No Cancer	6.2	+
17	No Cancer	6.2	+

18	No Cancer	7	+
19	No Cancer	10	+
20	No Cancer	10.4	+
21	Cancer	1.8	-
22	Cancer	2	-
23	Cancer	2	-
24	Cancer	2	-
25	Cancer	3	-
26	Cancer	3.8	-
27	Cancer	3.9	-
28	Cancer	4	-
29	Cancer	4.1	+

So, there are 20 patients who do not have cancer and 9 who do.
In the 20 patients who do not have cancer, 10 have a skin fold thickness less than or equal to 4mm and 10 have a skin fold thickness of more than 4 mm. In the 9 patients with cancer, 4 have a skin fold thickness equal to or less than 4 mm, whilst there is only 1 patient with a skin fold thickness more than 4 mm.

We can put this in a table:

	No Cancer	Cancer	Total
<= 4 mm	10	8	18
> 4 mm	10	1	11
Total	20	9	**29**

So, of the patients with cancer, there is only 1 out of 9 patients who has a skin thickness of more than 4 mm. Whilst 50% of the patients without cancer had a skin fold thickness of more than 4 mm. Is this due to chance or is there a statistically significant difference?

In chapter 2 we looked at probabilities. The probability of plus is 50% and the probability of minus is 50%.
If we test **two sided** we need to calculate the probability that:

P = 1 out of 9 patients > 4 mm + 0 out of 9 patients > 4 mm
        8 out of 9 patients < 4 mm + 9 out of 9 patients < 4 mm

So (chapter 2):

$$P = \binom{9}{1} * (0.5)^1 * (0.5)^8 + \binom{9}{0} * (0.5)^0 * (0.5)^9 +$$

$$\binom{9}{8} * (0.5)^8 * (0.5)^1 + \binom{9}{9} * (0.5)^9 * (0.5)^0$$

$$P = \frac{9!}{8!*1!} * (0.5) * (0.5)^8 + \frac{9!}{9!*0!} * (0.5)^9 +$$

$$\frac{9!}{1!*8!} * (0.5)^8 * (0.5) + \frac{9!}{0!*9!} * (0.5)^9$$

$$P = 9 * 0.001953125 + 1 * 0.001953125 + 9 * 0.001953125 + 1 * 0.001953125$$

$$P = 0.0390625$$

$P < 5\%$, therefore statistically significant.

Chi Square Test

In stead of the sign test, we use the Chi Square test as statistical test. Again we look at the table:

	No Cancer	Cancer	Total
<= 4 mm	10	8	18
> 4 mm	10	1	11
Total	20	9	**29**

In total, there were 18 out of 29 patients with a skin fold thickness <= 4mm.

If there were no difference between the two groups, we would expect:

$20 * \dfrac{18}{29}$ patients in the 'No Cancer' group and $9 * \dfrac{18}{29}$ patients in the 'Cancer' group with a skin thickness <= 4mm.

These are called the **expected frequencies**.

Similarly, we would expect:

$20 * \dfrac{11}{29}$ patients in the 'No Cancer' group and $9 * \dfrac{11}{29}$ patients in the 'Cancer' group with a skin thickness > 4mm.

If we list the expected frequencies in the table:

	No Cancer *Observed*	No Cancer *Expected*	Cancer *Observed*	Cancer *Expected*	Total
<= 4mm	10	12.4	8	5.6	18
>4 mm	10	7.6	1	3.4	11
Total	20	20	9	9	**29**

Now, using the Chi Square test we calculate:

$$\sum \frac{(O-E)^2}{E}$$ (O = Observed frequency and E = Expected frequency)

In our example:

$$\sum \frac{(O-E)^2}{E} = \frac{(10-12.4)^2}{12.4} + \frac{(8-5.6)^2}{5.6} + \frac{(10-7.6)^2}{7.6} + \frac{(1-3.4)^2}{3.4}$$

$\approx 0.469348659 + 1.04299702 + 0.768025078 + 1.706722396$

≈ 3.987093154

Next we need to determine the **degrees of freedom**:
In the observed frequencies table, there are two columns (c = 2) and two rows (r = 2). So there are (r - 1)*(c - 1) = 1 degree of freedom.

We can now look in a Chi Square distribution table (statistical table):

Degrees of Freedom	10%	5%	1%
1	2.71	3.84	6.63
2	4.61	5.99	9.21
3	6.25	7.81	11.34
4	7.78	9.49	13.28
5	9.24	11.07	15.09
10	15.99	18.31	23.21

Looking in the first row under one degree of freedom:

P = 3.84 at 5% and 6.63 at 1%.

3.987093154 > 3.84 and therefore the null hypothesis can be rejected in favour of the alternate hypothesis (p < 5%).
Please note that statistical significance is demonstrated at p <= 5%, but *not* at p <= 1%.

Mann Whitney U Test

Finally, we use the Mann-Whitney U test to analyse our data. The mathematics of this test is beyond the scope of this book. Suffice to say that the Mann Whitney U test is a rank test.
The data have been entered in a computer and analysed:

Mann-Whitney Rank Info for Skin Fold
Grouping Variable: Disease

	Count	Sum Ranks	Mean Rank
Cancer	9	91.500	10.167
No Cancer	20	343.500	17.175

In the table below, it can be seen that p < 5%, so again it is statistically significant:

Mann-Whitney U for Skin Fold
Grouping Variable: Disease

U	46.500
U Prime	133.500
Z-Value	-2.051
P-Value	.0403
Tied Z-Value	-2.053
Tied P-Value	.0401
# Ties	5

Which Statistical Test to Use?

There are many statistical tests described. So how do we know which test to use?
First of all we need to look at our data.
If the data are **not** continuous (chapter 3), we will have to use a non parametric test.

For nominal data (chapter 3), a frequency distribution such as the Chi Square test can be used.
When data are ordinal (can be ranked; chapter 3), it is usually better to use a rank test, such as the Mann Whitney U test.
The Mann Whitney U test can also be used for continuous data that are not normally distributed.

When data is continuous, we **might** be able to use a parametric test. However, we need to demonstrate that the data are normally distributed. This can be done with a test for normality, such as the Shapiro-Wilk test.
If the data has a normal distribution we can use parametric statistics. When the sample size is large (> 50), we can use the normal distribution as described above. For smaller sample sizes (< 50), the t-test is used.
We prefer to use a parametric test if possible, as these tests are more powerful (see below) than non parametric tests.

If the data are not normally distributed, we can not use a parametric test. In that case we could use, for example, the Mann Whitney U test.
If in doubt about the distribution of data (normal or not), we can always use a non parametric test. For example, we are allowed to use the Mann Whitney U test on normally distributed data (although it is less powerful). However, it is **incorrect** to use a t-test on data that is not normally distributed.

A summary is given in the table below:

Data	Sample Size	Test
Continuous	> 50	Normal
	< 50 Normal	t - Test
	< 50 Not Normal	Mann-Whitney U Test
Ordinal		Mann-Whitney U Test
Nominal		Chi - Squared Test

Obviously, there are many more tests described, but these are beyond the scope of this book.

Power of a Test

As stated above, we prefer to use parametric statistics if at all possible. Parametric tests are more **powerful** than non parametric tests. This means that we require fewer patients to demonstrate a statistically significant difference.
For example, (in analysing the same data) a t-test is more likely to demonstrate a statistically significant difference than a Mann Whitney U test. Similarly, the Mann Whitney U test is more powerful than the sign test.

Parametric tests are more powerful than non parametric tests because the distribution of the data is better known. If we know more about the distribution, we can incorporate this knowledge in our statistical test. The mathematics is not discussed here, but it appears logical that the more we know about the distribution, the more powerful a test can be.

If the test we use makes assumptions about the distribution of our data, we also limit its use to specific conditions. For example a t-test can only be used if data is normally distributed. So, in general, the more powerful a test, the more restricted its use.

Transformation of Data

In orthopaedics, data are often not normally distributed.
Occasionally however, data that are not normally distributed can be **transformed** to make the distribution normal. For example, by taking the logarithm or square our data. This process is called transformation of data. For example, the concentration of H_3O^+ in the peripheral blood is not normally distributed, but the pH ($-Log [H_3O^+]$) is.

Following transformation, it might be possible to use a more powerful parametric test (provided normality can be demonstrated).

As stated above, it is possible to use a non parametric test on parametric data. However, we can't use a parametric test on non parametric data. If we are in doubt about the distribution of our data, we can always use a non parametric test.

In analysing the outcome of hip replacements, functional scores (such as Harris hip score) are often used. They consist of a questionnaire that contains questions for pain, function and range of movement. A score is given for each category. They are added together and expressed as a percentage of normal function.

At first glance, the functional score obtained appears to be continuous data. So, provided normality can be demonstrated it seems reasonable to use a parametric test (such as the t-test).

However, when we look closer, the functional score is obtained by adding *ordinal* (chapter 3) data together (the answer to each question is given as a number, but in essence the data is ordinal). Hopefully it is obvious that by adding ordinal data together, the data remain ordinal and can never become continuous. Therefore, the data are not normally distributed and it is wrong to use a parametric test.

It also seems rather strange to add scores for function, pain and range of movement. These measures are completely different and should not be added together.

Summary Chapter 5

Null Hypothesis:	No difference between study groups
Alternate Hypothesis:	There is a difference between groups
Outcome Measure	Variable used to test the hypothesis
P Value	Probability that statement is incorrect
Statistically Significant	P < 5%
Parametric Test	Normal distribution
Non Parametric Test	Non normal distribution

Data	Sample Size	Test
Continuous	> 50	Normal
	< 50 Normal	t - Test
	< 50 Not Normal	Mann-Whitney U Test
Ordinal		Mann-Whitney U Test
Nominal		Chi - Squared Test

Questions Chapter 5

The table below shows the time to fracture healing (in weeks) in patients who presented with a tibial fracture. Smokers and non smokers are indicated in the second column:

Patient	Group	Time to Fracture Healing (Weeks)
1	Smoker	10
2	Smoker	11
3	Smoker	11
4	Smoker	12
5	Smoker	15
6	Smoker	17
7	Smoker	17
8	Smoker	18
9	Smoker	18
10	Smoker	19
11	Smoker	22
12	Smoker	24
13	Non Smoker	10
14	Non Smoker	10
15	Non Smoker	11
16	Non Smoker	12
17	Non Smoker	15
18	Non Smoker	15
19	Non Smoker	16
20	Non Smoker	17

1. Using the sign test and <=16 weeks as 'cut off' point; is fracture healing significantly delayed in patients who smoke? (significant when p < 5%)

2. Using the Chi Square test, is there a statistically significant difference? (significant when p < 5%). The Chi Square distribution table is shown below (same 'cut off' point; <= 16 weeks):

Degrees of Freedom	10%	5%	1%
1	2.71	3.84	6.63
2	4.61	5.99	9.21
3	6.25	7.81	11.34
4	7.78	9.49	13.28
5	9.24	11.07	15.09
10	15.99	18.31	23.21

Chapter 6 – Errors

When we have done our statistical test, we conclude whether the difference is statistically significant or not. Depending on that, we either accept or reject the null hypothesis. This decision could be correct or wrong.

We call α the probability of **rejecting the null hypothesis, when in fact it is true** (**false positive**). We usually set this significance level at 5%.

β is the probability of **incorrectly accepting the null hypothesis** (**false negative**).
The **power** (chapter 5) is the probability the test will **correctly reject the null hypothesis**. Therefore:

Power = 1 - β

We can make two types of errors:

Type 1 Error (or error of the first kind):
The null hypothesis is incorrectly rejected.
When the null hypothesis is rejected, we have concluded that there is a difference. However, this is incorrect (there really is no difference).
A type 1 error therefore, could be regarded as a **false positive**.
We can reduce the risk of a type one error by reducing the significance level (α).

Type 2 Error (or error of the second kind):
The null hypothesis is incorrectly accepted.
When the null hypothesis is accepted, we have concluded there is no difference. However, this is incorrect (there is a difference).
A type 2 error therefore, is a **false negative**. It is controlled with the Statistical Power (β)

We can reduce the probability of making a type 1 error by decreasing α (we usually set α at 5%). However, in doing so we increase the probability of making a type 2 error!

The graph below shows two normal distributions with a standard deviation of 0.5. The left curve has a mean of 0 and the right of 3:

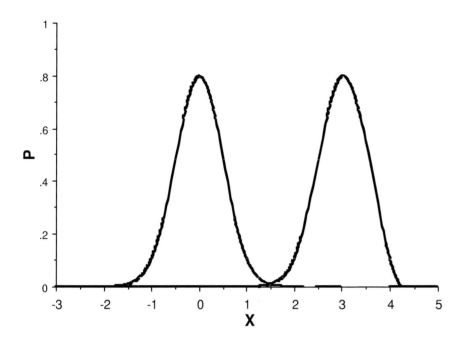

The graph below shows two normal distributions with a standard deviation of 2. The left curve has a mean of 0 and the right of 3:

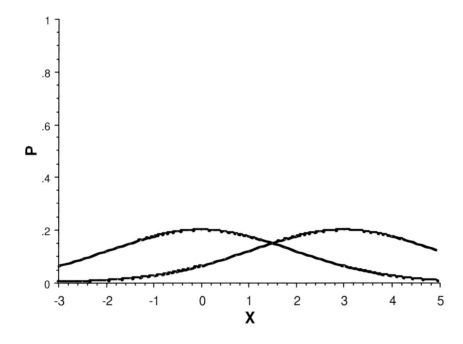

Looking at these graphs, it becomes obvious that errors are related to:

- **Difference desired to detect**

  If the difference in means is bigger (parametric statistics), we are less likely to commit an error.

  In non parametric statistics, we would look at the difference in mode.

- **Spread of data**

  The more the data are spread the more likely we are to commit an error. In parametric statistics this is indicated by a large standard deviation (or variance). Whilst in non parametric statistics, it is a larger range that demonstrates a bigger spread.

- **Significance level (α)**

  Selecting a lower significance level reduces the probability to commit a type 1 error. However, a type 2 error becomes more likely.

- **Test statistic (power)**

  By selecting a more powerful test (such as a parametric test), we are less likely to commit a type 2 error

Summary Chapter 6

α   **Probability of incorrectly rejecting the null hypothesis**
> **False positive**

β   **Probability of incorrectly accepting the null hypothesis**
> **False negative**

Power   **Probability of correctly rejecting the null hypothesis**
> **Power = 1 − β**

Errors:

Type 1   **Null hypothesis is incorrectly rejected**
> **False positive**
> **Significance level (α)**

Type 2   **Null hypothesis is incorrectly accepted**
> **False negative**
> **Statistical power**

Related to:

- **Difference desired to detect**
- **Spread of data**
- **Significance level (α)**
- **Test statistic (power)**

Chapter 7 – Sensitivity & Specificity

In medicine, we often use diagnostic tests to make a diagnosis. For example, we perform an MRI-scan to diagnose a meniscal tear or a CT-scan to see if someone has a tarsal coalition.

We all know that some diagnostic tests are better than others. An MRI-scan of the knee, for example, is better in diagnosing a meniscal tear than a CT scan, which in turn is better than a plain radiograph (*This of cause does **not** mean one should not request a radiograph of the knee when a meniscal tear is suspected. The radiograph is very helpful in eliminating other causes of knee pain or locking such as osteochondritis dissecans*). If one test is better than another in diagnosing a condition, we would like to know **how much better** this test is. To do this we can **validate** the test against a **gold standard**.

Five features of a diagnostic test have been described. These are **sensitivity, specificity, positive predictive value, negative predictive value** and **accuracy**. These five features allow us to **compare** different tests. They will be explained with an (made up) example.

As an example, we look at the value of MRI in diagnosing a meniscal tear in the knee. We need to **validate** the MRI against a **gold standard** (or the 'truth' as we perceive it). In this case, we use diagnostic arthroscopy as the gold standard. However, we could have used alternatives (such as open arthrotomy, which is obviously less acceptable nowadays).

In our example, we have 100 patients with a suspected meniscal tear. All patients had an MRI-scan that was reviewed by a radiologist. The radiologist reported the scan as either positive or negative for a meniscal tear. The radiologist was not allowed to be indecisive. After the patient had an MRI-scan, a diagnostic arthroscopy was performed. The orthopaedic surgeon, who performed the procedure, diagnosed a meniscal tear or not. Other pathology found by the orthopaedic surgeon, such as arthritis, is irrelevant in this context.

We are now going to validate the radiological diagnosis against the arthroscopic diagnosis. So, we assume that the arthroscopic diagnosis is always correct (surgeon is always right!).

There are 4 possible combinations:

a. The radiologist and orthopaedic surgeon both agree that there is a meniscal tear.
b. The radiologist diagnosed a meniscal tear but this was not confirmed at arthroscopy (*over diagnosis by radiologist*).
c. The radiologist reported the scan as normal, but there was a meniscal tear at arthroscopy (*missed diagnosis by radiologist*).
d. They both agree there is no meniscal tear.

We can put these four possibilities in a 2 * 2 table:

	Arthroscopy *positive*	**Arthroscopy** *negative*	
MRI *positive*	a	b	
MRI *negative*	c	d	

In this table, we have put the gold standard ('truth') in the columns and the test we validate against this standard in rows. It is important to realise that the formulas that follow will be different if we change this.

We are validating the result of the MRI-scan against the arthroscopic diagnosis. So, value **a** is the number of patients who have been correctly diagnosed as having a meniscal tear by MRI-scan. They are called the **True Positive** scans. Similarly, we can see that value **b** is the **False Positive**, value **c** the **False Negative**s and value **d** the **True Negative** scans. Or:

a. **True Positive**
b. **False Positive**
c. **False Negative**
d. **True Negative**

Next we will define the five features of a diagnostic test that have been described. These are:

a. Positive Predictive Value
b. Negative Predictive Value
c. Sensitivity
d. Specificity
e. Accuracy

Before we discuss these features, we will substitute the values of **a**, **b**, **c** and **d** with numbers:

	Arthroscopy positive	**Arthroscopy** negative	
MRI positive	49	5	
MRI negative	1	45	

In total there were 100 patients. So, a + b + c + d = 100:

	Arthroscopy positive	**Arthroscopy** negative	
MRI positive	49	5	
MRI negative	1	45	
			100

Positive Predictive Value

The positive predictive value of a test is defined as:

$$\frac{\text{True Positive who are also Test Positive}}{\text{All Test Positive}}$$

Or, in our example:

	Arthroscopy *positive*	Arthroscopy *negative*	
MRI *positive*	49	5	54
MRI *negative*	1	45	
			100

$$\frac{a}{(a+b)}$$

$$\frac{49}{(49+5)} = \frac{49}{(54)} = 0.907 \approx 91\%$$

So, 91% of the patients who had a positive MRI-scan were indeed found to have a meniscal tear at arthroscopy. 9% of the patients with a positive scan did not have a meniscal tear. Patients with a positive MRI-scan are therefore likely to have a meniscal tear (91%).
The positive predictive value is the probability that a person who is test positive indeed has the condition. The value ranges from 0 to 100 %.
If the positive predictive value is 100%, all test positives are also true positives. In other words, there will be no patients with a false positive test (b=0).
If the positive predictive value is 50%, there are as many true positives as there are false positives (a=b). Consequently, a positive test has no value in diagnosing disease.
If the positive predictive value is 0%, there are no true positives (a=0), and all people with a positive test are false positives. This does not necessarily mean that the test is useless. It might well be that a negative test is helpful in excluding disease.

Negative Predictive Value

The negative predictive value of a test is defined as:

$$\frac{\text{True Negative who are also Test Negative}}{\text{All Test Negative}}$$

Or, in our example:

	Arthroscopy *positive*	Arthroscopy *negative*	
MRI *positive*	49	5	54
MRI *negative*	1	45	46
			100

$$\frac{d}{(c+d)}$$

$$\frac{45}{(45+1)} = \frac{45}{(46)} = 0.978 \approx 98\%$$

So, 98% of the patients who had a negative MRI-scan indeed did not have a meniscal tear at arthroscopy. Only 2% of the patients with a negative scan were found to have a meniscal tear at arthroscopy. Patients with a negative MRI-scan are therefore unlikely to have a meniscal tear.
The negative predictive value is the probability that a person who is test negative does not have the condition. The value ranges from 0 to 100 %.
If the negative predictive value is 100%, all test negatives are also true negatives. In other words, there will be no patients with a false negative test (c=0).
If the negative predictive value is 50%, there are as many true negatives as there are false negatives (c=d). Consequently, a negative test has no value in excluding disease.
If the negative predictive value is 0%, there are no true negatives (d=0), and all people with a negative test are false negatives. This does not necessarily mean that the test is useless. It might well be that a positive test is helpful in diagnosing disease.

Sensitivity

The sensitivity of a test is defined as:

$$\frac{\text{True Positive who are also Test Positive}}{\text{All Positive}}$$

Or in our example:

	Arthroscopy *positive*	Arthroscopy *negative*	
MRI *positive*	49	5	54
MRI *negative*	1	45	46
	50		100

$$\frac{a}{(a+c)}$$

$$\frac{49}{(49+1)} = \frac{49}{(50)} = 0.98 = 98\%$$

So, 98% of the patients who were found to have a meniscal tear at arthroscopy had a positive MRI-scan. Only 2% of the patients with a meniscal tear had a negative MRI-scan. Therefore, an MRI-scan is very good in picking up patients who have a meniscal tear.
The sensitivity, or true positive rate, describes how good a test is in picking up people with the condition. The value ranges from 0 to 100 %. If the sensitivity is 100%, all positives are true positives. In other words, there are no false negatives (c=0).
If the sensitivity is 50%, there are as many true positives as there are false negatives (a=c). Indicating that the test has no use in picking up disease.
If the sensitivity is 0%, there are no true positives (a=0), and all people with the condition are false negatives. This does not necessarily mean the test is useless. It might well be good in excluding disease.

Specificity

The specificity of a test is defined as:

$$\frac{\text{True Negative who are also Test Negative}}{\text{All Negative}}$$

Or in our example:

	Arthroscopy *positive*	**Arthroscopy** *negative*	
MRI *positive*	49	5	54
MRI *negative*	1	45	46
	50	50	100

$$\frac{d}{(b+d)}$$

$$\frac{45}{(45+5)} = \frac{45}{(50)} = 0.9 = 90\%$$

So, 90% of the patients who (at arthroscopy) did not have a meniscal tear had a negative MRI-scan. 10% of the patients without a meniscal tear had a positive MRI-scan. Therefore, an MRI-scan is good in excluding patients who do not have a meniscal tear.
The specificity, or true negative rate, describes how good a test is in correctly excluding people without the condition. The value ranges from 0 to 100 %.
If the specificity is 100%, all negatives are true negatives. In other words, there are no false positives (b=0).
If the specificity is 50%, there are as many true negatives as there are false positives (b=d). Indicating that the test has no use in excluding disease.
If the specificity is 0%, there are no true negatives (d=0), and all people without the condition are false positives. This does not necessarily mean the test is useless. It might well be good in picking up disease.

Accuracy

The accuracy of a test is defined as:

Proportion of tests that have given the correct result
(true positives and true negatives).

Or, in our example:

	Arthroscopy *positive*	**Arthroscopy** *negative*	
MRI *positive*	49	5	54
MRI *negative*	1	45	46
	50	50	100

$$\frac{a+d}{(a+b+c+d)}$$

$$\frac{49+45}{(49+5+1+45)} = \frac{94}{(100)} = 94\%$$

So, in 94% of all MRI-scans performed, the result of the scan was correct. Accuracy 'combines' the specificity and the sensitivity of a test. The value is between 0 and 100 %.
If the accuracy of a test is 100%, there were no false positives and no false negatives (b=0 and c=0). Indicating that the test is very useful.
If the accuracy is 50%, there are just as many incorrect as correct results. In other words, the true positives plus true negatives equal the false positives plus false negatives (a+d = b+c). Consequently, the test is useless in diagnosing the disease.
If the accuracy is 0%, there are no true positives and true negatives (a=0 and d=0). Indicating that the test is always incorrect! This does not necessarily mean the test is useless. It could be just as useful to know if a test is incorrect as if it is correct.

Precision

Accuracy should not be confused with precision. Precision is something completely different. It is defined as the **closeness of repeated measurements of the same quantity.** Whilst accuracy is the closeness of a measured variate to its true value.

Precision indicates the variability of the estimate over all samples. A precise indicator will have a small variability (small standard deviation)

For example, let us consider a person with a mass of 65.2 kg.

We measure this person repeatedly on our scale and we find the mass 60.00001 kg (standard deviation 0.0000001). This is very precise, but not very accurate.

Repeatability

In this context, we should also mention repeatability.

If a measurement is repeated, we almost certainly get a different answer each time. If the variation is small, the repeatability is high.

Obviously, there is a difference if the measurement is repeated by the same person or another person. *Intra observer variation* is the variation that occurs when the same persons repeats the measurements. Whilst *Inter observer variation* is the variation that occurs when a different person repeats the measurements. We would normally expect the inter-observer variation to be larger than the intra-observer variation.

Validation

Validation is confirmation (by evidence) that the measure can be used consistently for its intended use.

For example, let us assume we have designed a machine that scans hand radiographs of children to calculate the bone age. Once we have collected a series of data, we need to confirm that we can use our machine to scan the bone age. We need to validate it against for example the Tanner-Whitehouse method.

In general:

	Truth *positive*	**Truth** *negative*	
Test *positive*	a	b	a + b
Test *negative*	c	d	c + d
	a + c	b + d	a + b + c + d

True Positive:	a
False Positive:	b
False Negative:	c
True Negative:	d

Positive Predictive Value: $\dfrac{a}{(a+b)}$

Negative Predictive Value: $\dfrac{d}{(c+d)}$

Sensitivity: $\dfrac{a}{(a+c)}$

Specificity: $\dfrac{d}{(b+d)}$

Accuracy: $\dfrac{a+d}{(a+b+c+d)}$

In the table, we have put the gold standard ('truth') in the columns and the test we validate against this standard in rows. It is important to realise that the formulas will be different if we change the columns and rows. It is therefore not advisable to learn the formulas of by heart. It is better to approach it systematically.

It should also be clear from the previous that any of the five parameters discussed **on their own** are of limited value. If one wants to look at just one parameter, the accuracy is the most informative.

However, it is better to look at the 4 * 4 table and calculate all parameters. This is further illustrated in the examples that follow.

Example 1:

Very sensitive test (fire alarm):

	Truth *positive*	**Truth** *negative*	
Test *positive*	1	39	40
Test *negative*	0	60	60
	1	99	100

True Positive:	1
False Positive:	39
False Negative:	0
True Negative:	60

Positive Predictive Value: $\dfrac{1}{40} = 2.5\%$

Negative Predictive Value: $\dfrac{60}{60} = 100\%$

Sensitivity: $\dfrac{1}{1} = 100\%$

Specificity: $\dfrac{60}{99} \approx 61\%$

Accuracy: $\dfrac{61}{100} = 61\%$

Example 2:

Very specific test (being caught for speeding):

	Truth *positive*	**Truth** *negative*	
Test *positive*	1	0	1
Test *negative*	39	60	99
	40	60	100

True Positive:	1
False Positive:	0
False Negative:	39
True Negative:	60

Positive Predictive Value: $\dfrac{1}{1} = 100\%$

Negative Predictive Value: $\dfrac{60}{99} \approx 61\%$

Sensitivity: $\dfrac{1}{40} = 2.5\%$

Specificity: $\dfrac{60}{60} = 100\%$

Accuracy: $\dfrac{61}{100} = 61\%$

It is important to bear in mind that a test can be sensitive for one purpose, but not necessarily for another.

For example, a bone scan is very sensitive in picking up abnormalities such as fractures and infections. However, it is not very helpful in picking up multiple myeloma. For that purpose, it would be better to use a bone marrow biopsy or MRI scan of the marrow areas.

If a test is used for screening, it is very important to make sure it has a high sensitivity. It is obviously unsatisfactory to miss disease with a screening investigation. If this investigation is not very specific, we can always perform further investigations to increase diagnostic accuracy (eliminate the false positives).

All tests have their limitations, and we should try to select the most appropriate investigation for what we are investigating. Sometimes we can use a combination of investigations. Usually, we start with the simplest and most sensitive investigations and increase diagnostic accuracy with more specific investigations.

Summary Chapter 7

Sensitivity (true +ve rate): **How good a test is in picking up people with the condition**

$$\frac{\text{True Positive who are also Test Positive}}{\text{All Positive}}$$

Specificity (true –ve rate): **How good a test is in excluding people without the condition**

$$\frac{\text{True Negative who are also Test Negative}}{\text{All Negative}}$$

Positive Predictive Value: **The probability that a person who is test positive indeed has the condition**

$$\frac{\text{True Positive who are also Test Positive}}{\text{All Test Positive}}$$

Negative Predictive Value: **The probability that a person who is test negative does not have the condition**

$$\frac{\text{True Negative who are also Test Negative}}{\text{All Test Negative}}$$

Accuracy: **Proportion of tests that have given the correct result**

Precision: **Closeness of repeated measurements of the same quantity**

	Truth *positive*	Truth *negative*	
Test *positive*	**a**	**b**	**a + b**
Test *negative*	**c**	**d**	**c + d**
	a + c	**b + d**	**a + b + c + d**

True Positive:	a
False Positive:	b
False Negative:	c
True Negative:	d

Positive Predictive Value: $\dfrac{a}{(a+b)}$

Negative Predictive Value: $\dfrac{d}{(c+d)}$

Sensitivity: $\dfrac{a}{(a+c)}$

Specificity: $\dfrac{d}{(b+d)}$

Accuracy: $\dfrac{a+d}{(a+b+c+d)}$

Questions Chapter 7

We are interested in evaluating the value of radioisotope bone scanning in the diagnosis of multiple myeloma.

We identified 50 consecutive patients who were suspected of having multiple myeloma and had a high erythrocyte sedimentation rate (>10 mm per hour).
All 50 patients had a radioisotope bone scan. Ten patients had a positive bone scan, showing one or more areas of increased uptake of radioisotope.

In 36 of these 50 patients the diagnosis of multiple myeloma was made following bone marrow aspiration. Six of these patients had a positive bone scan.

1.   Calculate the following parameters:

       True Positives
       True Negatives
       False Positives
       False Negatives

       Positive Predictive Value
       Negative Predictive Vale
       Sensitivity
       Specificity
       Accuracy

2.   On the basis of these parameters, is radioisotope bone scanning useful in making the diagnosis in patients with suspected multiple myeloma?

Chapter 8 – Curve Fitting

One often wants to know if there is a relation between two variables. To look if there is such a relation, an experiment can be designed. This experiment provides us data that can be plotted in a graph. Next, we will try to fit a line or curve that best fits these data. The mathematical equation of the curve gives us the relation.

Most commonly, one will try to fit a straight line through the data and this process is called linear curve fitting. Linear curve fitting is explained in the first part of this chapter.

It is however also possible to fit non-linear curves to data and this is explained in the second part of this chapter.

Linear Curve fitting

Linear curve fitting will be explained with an example.
We think there might be a relation between the girth and mass of a tree. The girth of 30 trees and their corresponding mass was measured. The data are shown in the table below:

Girth	Mass		Girth	Mass
205	251		327	693
213	272		327	737
219	335		334	610
226	278		343	733
231	375		347	673
241	335		351	726
250	410		358	760
266	414		358	788
266	478		360	766
275	560		362	750
296	489		362	737
299	506		363	707
314	606		368	821
315	616		369	827
321	562		372	772

As can be seen, we selected only trees with a girth between 200 and 375 centimetres. In this case, the girth is the *independent variable* and the mass the *dependent variable*.

If we had selected trees according to their mass rather than girth, the mass would have been the independent variable and the girth the dependent variable.

Next, we can plot the data in a graph. Customary, **the independent variable is plotted on the x-axis and the dependent variable on the y-axis:**

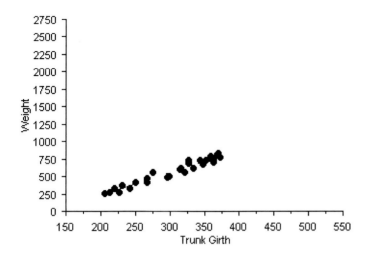

In linear curve fitting, we will try to draw a straight line that fits the data best. One way of doing this is to plot the data as shown above and draw a line through it with a ruler. When we draw the line, we will try to have as many data points above as below the line. This is certainly an acceptable method and seems to be no problem in the example above.
However, the data do not always lie close to a straight line. If they would lie further apart, it would be more difficult to draw a straight line through them. Furthermore, this graphical method is not very consistent.
A mathematical method is favoured as is far more consistent than a graphical method.

There are several mathematical methods described to fit a straight line through data points and full discussion of these is beyond the scope of this book. One method commonly used is the least square method. This is illustrated in the next graph:

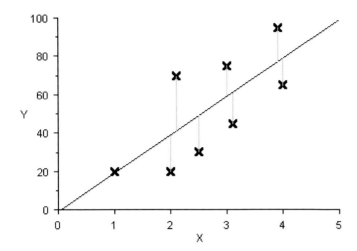

One imagines a straight line through the data. The distance of the dependent variable to this proposed line is calculated. Next the square of this distance is taken. This is done for two reasons:

- Points below the line have a negative distance and points above the line a positive distance. They therefore tend to cancel each other out. In taking the square, all distances become positive; eliminating the problem.
- By taking the square, data points further away from the proposed line are given more 'weight' than those close to the line.

This process is repeated for all straight lines possible. The best fitting line is that were the sum of the squares is **least**. This method is therefore called the **least square method**.

Nowadays, computers are used to perform these calculations.

Regression Coefficient

A straight line has the following basic equation:

$$y = a*x + b$$

Were x is the independent variable and y the dependent variable.
'a' is the ***regression coefficient***. It represents the slope of the line and can be calculated by dividing the difference in y-value to the difference in x-value at two points:

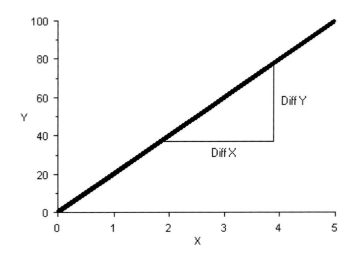

If a = 0, the line is horizontal. The larger the value of 'a', the more vertical (steeper) the line is:

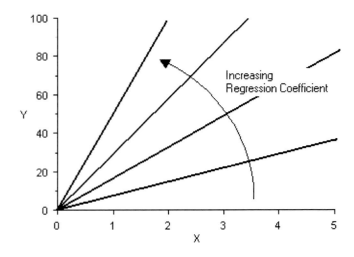

A negative value of 'a' corresponds to a downwards slope:

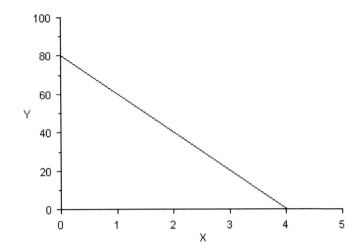

In the graph above, the regression coefficient = - 20 $\left(\dfrac{80}{-4}\right)$.

'b' is a constant for the line and represents the y-value at x = 0.
If the line goes through the origin of the coordinate system (0,0), than b = 0.
If the line crosses above the origin, 'b' is positive and if it crosses below the origin, 'b' is negative. In the graph above, b = 80.
So:

Y = -20*x +80

We return to our tree example.
The computer has drawn the best fitting line through the data points using the least square method:

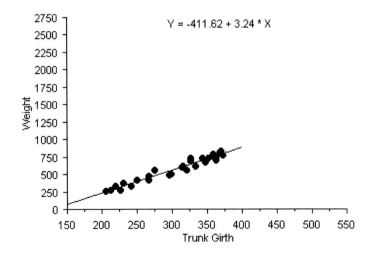

It can be seen that the regression coefficient is 3.24 and the value of b = -411.62.

The regression coefficient is a measure of the slope of the line. It ranges from -∞ to +∞. A regression coefficient of zero means the line is horizontal; a positive value corresponds to an upward slope and a negative value to a downward slope. The larger the value of the regression coefficient, the steeper the slope.

Correlation Coefficient

In our tree example, we have now fitted the best line through the data points. As can be seen in the graph, the line seems to fit the data well. However, this is not always the case.

One would like to have a measure of how close the line fits the data. This measure is called the ***correlation coefficient*** and often denoted by ***r***. It is defined as:

$$r = \frac{\text{Sum of Products about the Mean of X and Y}}{\sqrt{\text{Sum of Squares about the Mean of X times Sum of Squares about the Mean of Y}}}$$

Obviously, computers are commonly used to calculate the correlation coefficient.

In our tree example, the computer has calculated the correlation coefficient:

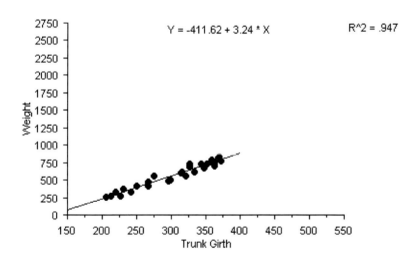

Calculation of the correlation coefficient involves taking the square root. Therefore, the squared correlation coefficient is often calculated. The correlation coefficient is found by taking the square root from this value. In our example, the correlation coefficient is $\sqrt{0.947} = 0.97$.

The correlation coefficient always has a value between −1 and 1. A correlation coefficient of 0.97 therefore, means that there is an excellent correlation between the girth and mass of a tree.

It should be noted that the square of the correlation coefficient is always **smaller** than the correlation coefficient itself. This is because the square of a number between −1 and 1 is always **smaller** than the number itself.

If the correlation coefficient = 1, the line fits the data perfectly:

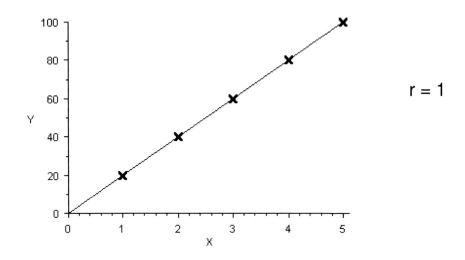

$$r = 1$$

A correlation coefficient of zero, means that there is no correlation whatsoever:

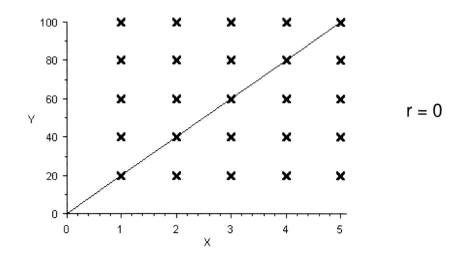

$$r = 0$$

In fact, we could have drawn **any line** through the data points above!
A correlation coefficient of −1, means that there is reverse relation between the data:

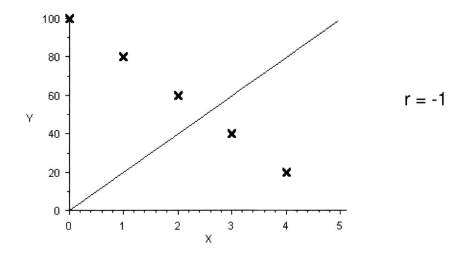

r = -1

The correlation coefficient is a measure how close the line fits the data. It ranges from −1 to +1. A correlation coefficient of zero means that there is no correlation. The more the value approaches 1, the better the line fits the data. A negative value corresponds to a reverse relation.

Interpolation

We have now found the equation of the line showing the relation between girth and mass of a tree. In our example, we had to chop the tree down in order to measure its mass.
We would now like to use the equation to estimate the mass of a tree by only measuring its girth; without chopping it down!
From the equation we can estimate the mass of a tree with a girth of 280 centimetres:

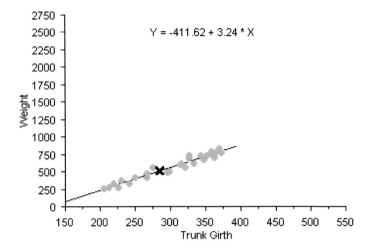

Mass = -411.62 + 3.24 * 280

Mass = 495.58 kilogram

The estimation we made is ***within the range we have measured***. This process is called interpolation.

Extrapolation

Similarly, we can estimate the mass of a tree ***outside the range we have measured***. This process is called extrapolation:

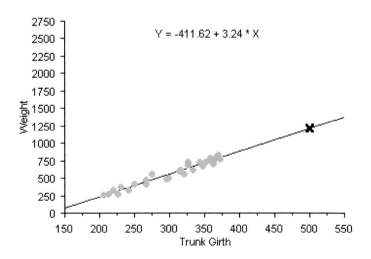

In our example, we can estimate the mass of a tree with a girth of 500 centimetres as:

Mass = -411.62 + 3.24*500
Mass = 1208.38 kilogram

Obviously, one has to be far more cautious with estimations found by means of extrapolation than with interpolation.

Non-Linear Curve Fitting

In our tree example, we only looked at trees with a girth between 200 and 375 centimetres. We also extrapolated our data and calculated that a tree with a diameter of 500 centimetres would have a mass of 1208 kilogram. It has been stated above that one should be cautious in extrapolating data. To demonstrate this we have slightly extended our experiment.

We have now measured 104 trees with a girth between 0 and 550 centimetres. There measurements are as follows:

Girth	Weight	Girth	Weight	Girth	Weight	Girth	Weight
205	251	369	827	410	1035	460	1751
213	272	372	772	412	1418	463	1556
219	335	375	821	412	1412	463	1838
226	278	375	790	414	1167	464	1455
231	375	376	912	416	1151	464	1937
241	335	376	800	421	1326	465	1244
250	410	380	885	424	1392	465	1658
266	414	381	882	424	1177	467	1613
266	478	382	1052	425	1488	469	1495
275	560	385	1017	427	1242	469	1490
296	489	387	1052	428	1176	473	1817
299	506	387	981	431	1609	478	1571
314	606	389	944	435	1304	479	1381
315	616	390	944	438	1197	482	1331
321	562	392	1067	438	1197	484	1789
327	693	393	928	440	1026	487	1635
327	737	394	1009	441	1137	498	1517
334	610	395	1085	442	1242	514	2266
343	733	395	952	444	1398	522	2508
347	673	398	1209	448	1475	527	2375
351	726	399	853	448	1258		
358	760	401	1012	450	1288		
358	788	404	1084	451	1290		
360	766	405	1241	452	1499		
362	750	405	1023	456	1458		
362	737	406	1094	457	1506		
363	707	408	1149	457	1325		
368	821	409	1036	457	1823		

If we plot the data in a graph and draw the best fitting line using the least square method, the graph will be as follows:

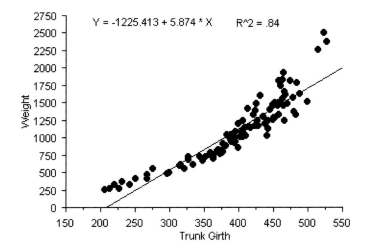

As can be seen from the graph, this line does not appear to fit as well to this extended data set as it did previously. This is also reflected in the correlation coefficient, which is:

$$\sqrt{0.84} \quad = 0.92.$$

Although, the correlation coefficient is still pretty good, it is not as good as it was before.

Closer examination of the data shows not a linear, but perhaps an exponential relation.
We can try to fit such an exponential curve with the standard equation

$$Y = b * e^{(a * X)}$$

through our data.

The mathematics of this are beyond the scope of this book. If we fit an exponential curve through our data using the computer we get the following graph:

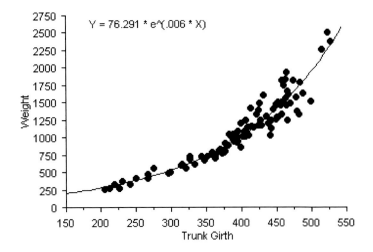

It can be seen that the curve fits the data much better. If we think about it, an exponential relation appears more logical than a linear relation between girth and mass of a tree.

We can now calculate the mass of a tree with a girth of 500 centimetres again using our new formula:

$$Y = 76.291 * e^{(0.006 * X)}$$

We get:

$$Mass = 76.291 * e^{(0.006 * 500)} = 1532.35 \text{ kilogram.}$$

This is considerable more than the 1208 kilogram we calculated with extrapolation of a straight line. If we look at our graph, we can see that a value of 1532 kilogram appears to be more realistic.
This example highlights the dangers of extrapolating data.

Summary Chapter 8

- **The independent variable is plotted on the x-axis and the dependent variable on the y-axis**

- **The regression coefficient is a measure of the slope of the line. It ranges from -∞ to +∞. A regression coefficient of zero means the line is horizontal; a positive value corresponds to an upward slope and a negative value to a downward slope. The larger the value the steeper the slope**

- **The correlation coefficient is a measure how close the line fits the data. It ranges from −1 to +1. A correlation coefficient of zero means that there is no correlation. The more the value approaches 1, the better the line fits the data. A negative value corresponds to a reverse relation**

- **Interpolation is estimation of a non-measured value *within* the range that has been measured**

- **Extrapolation is estimation of a non-measured value *outside* the range that has been measured**

- **One has to be cautious extrapolating data**

Questions Chapter 8

Consider the following data set:

X	Y
3	1.2
4	1.4
5	1.6
6	1.75
7	1.85

1.
    a. Plot the data in a graph.
    b. Draw the best fitting line through the data points using the graphical method.
    c. From the graph, estimate the equation of the line.
2. Estimate the correlation coefficient.
3. Interpolate the value for x = 5.5.
4. Extrapolate the value for x = 0.1 and x = 15.

Consider the extended data set below:

X	Y
0.1	-1.25
0.2	-0.7
1	0.4
2	0.9
3	1.2
4	1.4
5	1.6
6	1.75
7	1.85
8	1.95
9	2.05
10	2.1
12	2.25
14	2.35
15	2.4

5. Plot these data in a graph
6. What is the relation between x and y and what is the value of the correlation coefficient?
7. What are the y-values for x = 0.1 and x = 15?

Chapter 9 – Survival Analysis

As the name implies, survival analysis was developed to analyse the survival of cancer patients. It estimates the probability of survival after a period of time.

The probability of survival can be calculated at yearly intervals. With these figures, a survival curve can be constructed.

Survival analysis is very useful as it allows comparison of survival of patients treated by different methods (chemotherapeutic regimes).

Survival analysis calculates the probability of survival of a group of patients between two events, the start date and the end date. The start date is normally date of diagnosis or date of surgery. The end is the date of failure.

It is very important to define what failure is. One can define death as failure and being alive as success. In that case, we have defined a 'hard end point'; we cannot argue about the outcome.

However, survival analysis has been extended beyond estimating survival rates in cancer patients. It is also been used to estimate survival of total joint replacements. In this case, it is not so easy to define a 'hard end point'. Later, we will discuss the implications of an end point that is not 'hard' in more detail.

For now it is important to realise that:

In survival analysis it is essential to define a 'hard end point' for the event of interest.

There are several methods to perform survival analysis. The most elementary method is life table survival analysis. Another method is Kaplan-Meier survival analysis, which will be discussed later in this chapter. We will start with life table analysis.

Life Table Survival Analysis

It is easiest to explain **life table survival analysis** with an example. We look at 10 patients who have been diagnosed with cancer. The date of diagnosis is shown in the 2nd column of the table below. Analysis was performed on 1/2/2001.

Patients who were alive at 1/2/2001, had this date inserted in the 3rd column (date last follow up). If the patient died, the date of death was inserted in the 3rd column. The 4th column indicates which patients died and which patients were alive:

Patient Number	Date Diagnosis	Date Last FU or †	Outcome
1	17/01/97	01/02/01	Alive
2	18/05/97	28/09/99	**Died**
3	18/09/97	25/01/99	**Died**
4	18/12/97	01/02/01	Alive
5	19/01/98	01/02/01	Alive
6	18/06/98	31/05/00	**Died**
7	18/10/98	01/02/01	Alive
8	18/02/99	01/02/01	Alive
9	18/08/99	01/02/01	Alive
10	18/12/99	01/02/01	Alive

We can also show the data in a graph:

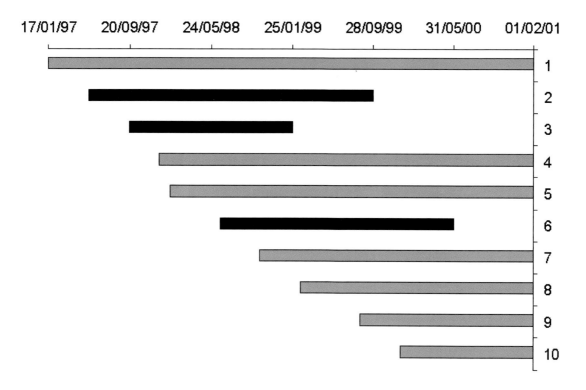

Patients who died are indicated in black and survivors in grey.

We now calculate the follow up between the two events (date of diagnosis and date of death / last follow up) for every patient::

Patient Number	Date Diagnosis	Date Last FU or †	FU (Years)	Outcome
1	17/01/97	01/02/01	4.04	Alive
2	18/05/97	28/09/99	2.34	**Died**
3	18/09/97	25/01/99	1.35	**Died**
4	18/12/97	01/02/01	3.12	Alive
5	19/01/98	01/02/01	3.04	Alive
6	18/06/98	31/05/00	1.95	**Died**
7	18/10/98	01/02/01	2.29	Alive
8	18/02/99	01/02/01	1.95	Alive
9	18/08/99	01/02/01	1.46	Alive
10	18/12/99	01/02/01	1.13	Alive

In total, we have 10 patients. All these patients have a follow up between 0 and 5 years. However, some patients have a follow up that is longer than others. We have to take this into account if we want to calculate the probability of survival.

We are now going to calculate the probability of survival at **yearly intervals** (see table below). We started with 10 patients. Therefore, there were 10 patients at the beginning of year 1.

From the table we can see that all patients had a follow up of more than 1 year. Therefore, at the start of the 2nd year there were still 10 patients.

Five patients had a follow up between 1 and 2 years. Two of these patients died and 3 patients were still alive at review. The 3 patients who were still alive have only been observed for **part** of the second year. They could still die during the remainder of that year. These 3 patients are called **withdrawn from follow up**.

Patients who have been withdrawn from follow up are also called **'censored'**; in other words the event of interest (death) was not observed. Similarly, patients are called **'uncensored'** if the event of interest (death) was observed. So, in the 2nd year, 2 patients were *uncensored* and 3 patients were *censored*.

At the beginning of the 3rd year there were 5 patients left. 2 patients had a follow up between 2 and 3 years. One of these patients died (uncensored) and 1 patient withdrew from follow up (censored).

Consequently, at the start of the 4th year there were only 3 patients left. 2 patients withdrew from follow up during the 4th year and none died.

This left only 1 patient at the start of year 5. This patient had a follow up of just over 4 years and consequently withdrew during the 5th year.

All these figures have been inserted in the table below:

Year	FU (Years)	No Patients @ Start Year	Withdrawn (Censored)	Died (Failure)
1	>0 & ≤1	10	0	0
2	>1 & ≤ 2	10	3	2
3	>2 & ≤ 3	5	1	1
4	>3 & ≤ 4	3	2	0
5	>4 & ≤ 5	1	1	0
6	>5 & ≤ 6	0	0	0

It must be clear that the number of patients at the start of a year, minus the patients withdrawn in that year minus the patients who died in that year make up the number of patients at the start of the next year. In other words: the number of patients at the start of a year minus the number **censored** minus the number **uncensored** in that year equals the number at the start of the next year.

For example, at the first year: there were 10 patients at the start, minus 0 patients who withdrew, minus 0 patients who died in that year. This equals 10 patients at the start of year 2.

Or:

$$10 - 0 - 0 = 10$$

Similarly, for the 2nd year:

$$10 - 3 - 2 = 5$$

And the 3rd year:

$$5 - 1 - 1 = 3$$

For the 4th year:

$$3 - 2 - 0 = 1$$

And the 5th year:

$$1 - 1 = 0$$

Patients who withdrew from follow up were observed for only part of that year. We know that they were alive at the date of last follow up and that the event of interest (death) has not occurred. However, there is a possibility that these patients might still die during the remainder of that year. We just don't have enough follow up to be sure. So, these patients are only at risk of death for part of that year. In other words: **the censored patients are at risk of the event of interest for only part of that year**. On average, these patients will only have half the risk.

In the first year, no patients withdrew from follow up. Therefore, we will start with the 2nd year. In that year 3 patients withdrew from follow up. These 3 patients have only been at risk for half of the 2nd year. We can say that only 1.5 of these patients have been at risk of death.

So, in total 8.5 patients (10 – 1.5) have been at risk of death during the 2nd year. This has been indicated in the 6th column in the table below.

Similarly, 4.5 patients (5 – 0.5) were at risk in the 3rd year, 2 (3 – 1) in the 4th year, 0.5 (1 – 0.5) in the 5th year and 0 in the last year:

Year	FU (Years)	No Patients @ Start Year	Withdrawn (Censored)	Died (Failure)	At Risk
1	>0 & ≤1	10	0	0	10
2	>1 & ≤ 2	10	3	2	8.5
3	>2 & ≤ 3	5	1	1	4.5
4	>3 & ≤ 4	3	2	0	2
5	>4 & ≤ 5	1	1	0	0.5
6	>5 & ≤ 6	0	0	0	0

As we have seen in chapter 2, the probability of the event of interest (death) equals:

$$\text{Probability (Failure)} = \frac{\text{Number of Patients Died}}{\text{Number of Patients at Risk}}$$

The probability of failure (death) has been calculated at yearly intervals and is indicated in the 7th column of the table below:

Year	FU (Years)	No Patients @ Start Year	Withdrawn (Censored)	Died (Failure)	At Risk	Probability of Failure
1	>0 & ≤1	10	0	0	10	0
2	>1 & ≤ 2	10	3	2	8.5	$\dfrac{2}{8.5}$
3	>2 & ≤ 3	5	1	1	4.5	$\dfrac{1}{4.5}$
4	>3 & ≤ 4	3	2	0	2	0
5	>4 & ≤ 5	1	1	0	0.5	0
6	>5 & ≤ 6	0	0	0	0	0

The probability of survival is:

Probability (Survival) = 1 – Probability (Failure)

The probability of success (survival) has been calculated at yearly intervals and is shown in the 8th column in the table below:

Year	FU (Years)	No Patients @ Start Year	Withdrawn (Censored)	Died (Failure)	At Risk	Probability of Failure	Probability of Survival
1	>0 & ≤1	10	0	0	10	0	1
2	>1 & ≤ 2	10	3	2	8.5	$\dfrac{2}{8.5}$	$\dfrac{6.5}{8.5}$
3	>2 & ≤ 3	5	1	1	4.5	$\dfrac{1}{4.5}$	$\dfrac{3.5}{4.5}$
4	>3 & ≤ 4	3	2	0	2	0	1
5	>4 & ≤ 5	1	1	0	0.5	0	1
6	>5 & ≤ 6	0	0	0	0	0	

The probability of surviving two years obviously depends on having survived the first year. Similarly, the probability on surviving 3 years depends on having survived year 1 and 2; and so on. As we discussed in chapter 2 these dependent probabilities should be multiplied.

We are therefore interested in the **cumulative survival**. Being a probability, the cumulative survival is a figure between 0 and 1 (or 0% and 100%).

In our example the probability of surviving the 1st year is 1, the probability of surviving the 2nd year $1*\dfrac{6.5}{8.5}$, the third year $1*\dfrac{6.5}{8.5}*\dfrac{3.5}{4.5}$, the 4th year $1*\dfrac{6.5}{8.5}*\dfrac{3.5}{4.5}*1$ and $1*\dfrac{6.5}{8.5}*\dfrac{3.5}{4.5}*1*1$ the 5th year.

The cumulative survival in our example is shown in the last column of the table below:

Year	FU (Years)	No Patients @ Start Year	Withdrawn (Censored)	Died (Failure)	At Risk	Prob of Survival	Cumulative Survival
1	>0 & ≤1	10	0	0	10	1	1
2	>1 & ≤ 2	10	3	2	8.5	$\dfrac{6.5}{8.5}$	$1*\dfrac{6.5}{8.5}$
3	>2 & ≤ 3	5	1	1	4.5	$\dfrac{3.5}{4.5}$	$1*\dfrac{6.5}{8.5}*\dfrac{3.5}{4.5}$
4	>3 & ≤ 4	3	2	0	2	1	$1*\dfrac{6.5}{8.5}*\dfrac{3.5}{4.5}*1$
5	>4 & ≤ 5	1	1	0	0.5	1	$1*\dfrac{6.5}{8.5}*\dfrac{3.5}{4.5}*1*1$
6	>5 & ≤ 6	0	0	0	0		

If we perform the calculation:

Year	FU (Years)	No Patients @ Start Year	Withdrawn (Censored)	Died (Failure)	At Risk	Prob of Survival	Cumulative Survival
1	>0 & ≤1	10	0	0	10	1	**1**
2	>1 & ≤ 2	10	3	2	8.5	$\dfrac{6.5}{8.5}$	**0.765**
3	>2 & ≤ 3	5	1	1	4.5	$\dfrac{3.5}{4.5}$	**0.595**
4	>3 & ≤ 4	3	2	0	2	1	**0.595**
5	>4 & ≤ 5	1	1	0	0.5	1	**0.595**
6	>5 & ≤ 6	0	0	0	0		

Or in percentages:

Year	FU (Years)	No Patients @ Start Year	Withdrawn (Censored)	Died (Failure)	At Risk	Prob of Survival	Cumulative Survival (%)
1	>0 & ≤1	10	0	0	10	1	100
2	>1 & ≤ 2	10	3	2	8.5	$\dfrac{6.5}{8.5}$	76.5
3	>2 & ≤ 3	5	1	1	4.5	$\dfrac{3.5}{4.5}$	59.5
4	>3 & ≤ 4	3	2	0	2	1	59.5
5	>4 & ≤ 5	1	1	0	0.5	1	59.5
6	>5 & ≤ 6	0	0	0	0		

The cumulative survival can also be plotted in a graph, as shown below.

To indicate that the survival has been calculated at *yearly intervals*, the graph is *stepped* rather than smooth.

The survival curve is stepped at yearly intervals in life table survival analysis:

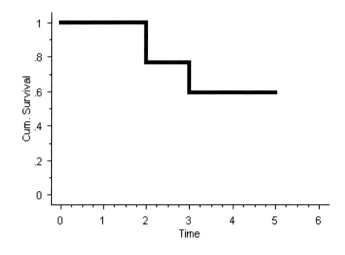

In our example, all patients who did not die were reviewed on 1st February 2001. In reality however, we often have patients who were lost to follow up. So how do we deal with this situation?

We will look at our example again, but now assume that the patients with number 5,7 and 10 were lost to follow up. The last time they were seen was on 31st May 2000. At that time they were alive and well. What happened after is not known. This is indicated in the table below:

Patient Number	Date Diagnosis	Date Last FU or †	FU (Years)	Outcome
1	17/01/97	01/02/01	4.04	Alive
2	18/05/97	28/09/99	2.34	**Died**
3	18/09/97	25/01/99	1.35	**Died**
4	18/12/97	01/02/01	3.12	Alive
5	19/01/98	31/05/00	2.36	Lost to FU
6	18/06/98	31/05/00	1.95	**Died**
7	18/10/98	31/05/00	1.62	Lost to FU
8	18/02/99	01/02/01	1.95	Alive
9	18/08/99	01/02/01	1.46	Alive
10	18/12/99	31/05/00	0.45	Lost to FU

As before, we can now construct a table that shows the number of patients at the start of each year, the number of patients who withdrew (censored) and the patients who died (uncensored):

Year	FU (Years)	No Patients @ Start Year	Withdrawn (Censored)	Died (Failure)
1	>0 & ≤1	10	1	0
2	>1 & ≤ 2	9	3	2
3	>2 & ≤ 3	4	1	1
4	>3 & ≤ 4	2	1	0
5	>4 & ≤ 5	1	1	0
6	>5 & ≤ 6	0	0	0

The censored patients are only at risk for part of the year. On average, they will have half the risk.

The number of patients at risk per year has been calculated and is indicated in the 6th column of the table below:

Year	FU (Years)	No Patients @ Start Year	Withdrawn (Censored)	Died (Failure)	At Risk
1	>0 & ≤1	10	1	0	9.5
2	>1 & ≤ 2	9	3	2	7.5
3	>2 & ≤ 3	4	1	1	3.5
4	>3 & ≤ 4	2	1	0	1.5
5	>4 & ≤ 5	1	1	0	0.5
6	>5 & ≤ 6	0	0	0	0

As before, we can calculate the probability of failure, probability of survival and the cumulative survival:

Year	FU (Years)	No @ Start	Withdrawn (Censored)	Died (Failure)	At Risk	Prob of Failure	Prob of Survival	Cumulative Survival
1	>0 & ≤1	10	1	0	9.5	0	1	1
2	>1 & ≤ 2	9	3	2	7.5	$\frac{2}{7.5}$	$\frac{5.5}{7.5}$	$1*\frac{5.5}{7.5}$
3	>2 & ≤ 3	4	1	1	3.5	$\frac{1}{3.5}$	$\frac{2.5}{3.5}$	$1*\frac{5.5}{7.5}*\frac{2.5}{3.5}$
4	>3 & ≤ 4	2	1	0	1.5	0	1	$1*\frac{5.5}{7.5}*\frac{2.5}{3.5}*1$
5	>4 & ≤ 5	1	1	0	0.5	0	1	$1*\frac{5.5}{7.5}*\frac{2.5}{3.5}*1*1$
6	>5 & ≤ 6	0	0	0	0	0		

Or in percentages:

Year	FU (Years)	No @ Start	Withdrawn (Censored)	Died (Failure)	At Risk	Prob of Failure	Prob of Survival	Cumulative Survival (%)
1	>0 & ≤1	10	1	0	9.5	0	1	1
2	>1 & ≤ 2	9	3	2	7.5	$\dfrac{2}{7.5}$	$\dfrac{5.5}{7.5}$	73.3
3	>2 & ≤ 3	4	1	1	3.5	$\dfrac{1}{3.5}$	$\dfrac{2.5}{3.5}$	52.4
4	>3 & ≤ 4	2	1	0	1.5	0	1	52.4
5	>4 & ≤ 5	1	1	0	0.5	0	1	52.4
6	>5 & ≤ 6	0	0	0	0			

So, the cumulative survival at 5 years is 52%, which is almost the same as calculated previously (60%). However, we have counted the patients lost to follow up as **censored**. In doing so, we have counted them as a success! It is however possible that these patients have died. We just don't know (as they are lost to follow up). All we know is that they were alive on the 31st May 2000. They could have died the following day.

What we have calculated is the cumulative survival at 5 years, whilst the 3 patients lost to follow up have been counted as a success. In other words, we have calculated the **best-case scenario**.

So what is the **worst-case scenario**, when all patients lost to follow up are counted as failures (dead)?

We go back to our table:

Patient Number	Date Diagnosis	Date Last FU or †	FU (Years)	Outcome
1	17/01/97	01/02/01	4.04	Alive
2	18/05/97	28/09/99	2.34	**Died**
3	18/09/97	25/01/99	1.35	**Died**
4	18/12/97	01/02/01	3.12	Alive
5	19/01/98	31/05/00	2.36	Lost to FU
6	18/06/98	31/05/00	1.95	**Died**
7	18/10/98	31/05/00	1.62	Lost to FU
8	18/02/99	01/02/01	1.95	Alive
9	18/08/99	01/02/01	1.46	Alive
10	18/12/99	31/05/00	0.45	Lost to FU

This time we count the patients lost to follow up as having died:

Year	FU (Years)	No Patients @ Start Year	Withdrawn (Censored)	Died (Failure)
1	>0 & ≤1	10	0	1
2	>1 & ≤ 2	9	2	3
3	>2 & ≤ 3	4	0	2
4	>3 & ≤ 4	2	1	0
5	>4 & ≤ 5	1	1	0
6	>5 & ≤ 6	0	0	0

As before, we can calculate the number of patients at risk:

Year	FU (Years)	No Patients @ Start Year	Withdrawn (Censored)	Died (Failure)	At Risk
1	>0 & ≤1	10	0	1	10
2	>1 & ≤ 2	9	2	3	8
3	>2 & ≤ 3	4	0	2	4
4	>3 & ≤ 4	2	1	0	1.5
5	>4 & ≤ 5	1	1	0	0.5
6	>5 & ≤ 6	0	0	0	0

The probability of failure, probability of survival and cumulative survival have also been calculated and are indicated in the table below:

Year	FU (Years)	No @ Start	Withdrawn (Censored)	Died (Failure)	At Risk	Prob of Failure	Prob of Survival	Cumulative Survival
1	>0 & ≤1	10	0	1	10	$\frac{1}{10}$	$\frac{9}{10}$	$\frac{9}{10}$
2	>1 & ≤ 2	9	2	3	8	$\frac{3}{8}$	$\frac{5}{8}$	$\frac{9}{10}*\frac{5}{8}$
3	>2 & ≤ 3	4	0	2	4	$\frac{2}{4}$	$\frac{2}{4}$	$\frac{9}{10}*\frac{5}{8}*\frac{2}{4}$
4	>3 & ≤ 4	2	1	0	1.5	0	1	$\frac{9}{10}*\frac{5}{8}*\frac{2}{4}*1$
5	>4 & ≤ 5	1	1	0	0.5	0	1	$\frac{9}{10}*\frac{5}{8}*\frac{2}{4}*1*1$
6	>5 & ≤ 6	0	0	0	0	0		

Or in percentages:

Year	FU (Years)	No @ Start	Withdrawn (Censored)	Died (Failure)	At Risk	Prob of Failure	Prob of Survival	Cumulative Survival (%)
1	>0 & ≤1	10	0	1	10	$\dfrac{1}{10}$	$\dfrac{9}{10}$	90
2	>1 & ≤ 2	9	2	3	8	$\dfrac{3}{8}$	$\dfrac{5}{8}$	56.3
3	>2 & ≤ 3	4	0	2	4	$\dfrac{2}{4}$	$\dfrac{2}{4}$	28.1
4	>3 & ≤ 4	2	1	0	1.5	0	1	28.1
5	>4 & ≤ 5	1	1	0	0.5	0	1	28.1
6	>5 & ≤ 6	0	0	0	0	0		

So, we have now calculated the **best-case scenario** and the **worst-case scenario**. The cumulative survival at 5 years is at best 52% and at worst 28%. The reality is probably somewhere in between these two values.

We can also show the survival curves for **best-** and **worst-case scenarios** in a graph:

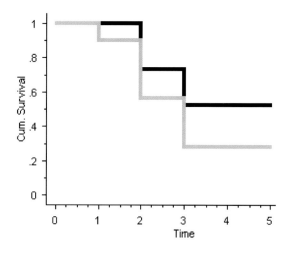

The **best-case scenario** is indicated in black and the **worst-case scenario** in grey.

So, **patients who are censored are either lost to follow up, or the event of interest has not yet occurred.** For patients who are lost to follow up, worse- and best-case scenarios can be calculated. In reality, the cumulative survival probably lies somewhere in between these two extremes.

Kaplan-Meier Survival Analysis

Apart from **life table analysis**, there are other methods of estimating the survival. One other method commonly used in medicine is the **Kaplan-Meier**, or product limit, survival analysis.

In Kaplan-Meier analysis, the probability of survival is not calculated at yearly intervals. Instead it is calculated from patient to patient. It is therefore necessary to rank the patients and create a table calculating the probability of survival. In general, Kaplan-Meier analysis is the preferred method of calculating survival. Again this is best explained with an example.

We will use the same example as we used before. This time we will perform a **Kaplan-Meier** (product limit) analysis on these data. The patients that are lost to follow up will be counted as a success. So, we will again be calculating the **best-case scenario**.

The table of are previous example is again show below:

Patient Number	Date Diagnosis	Date Last FU or †	FU (Years)	Outcome
1	17/01/97	01/02/01	4.04	Alive
2	18/05/97	28/09/99	2.34	**Died**
3	18/09/97	25/01/99	1.35	**Died**
4	18/12/97	01/02/01	3.12	Alive
5	19/01/98	31/05/00	2.36	Lost to FU
6	18/06/98	31/05/00	1.95	**Died**
7	18/10/98	31/05/00	1.62	Lost to FU
8	18/02/99	01/02/01	1.95	Alive
9	18/08/99	01/02/01	1.46	Alive
10	18/12/99	31/05/00	0.45	Lost to FU

We first rank the patients according to the **follow up.**

The columns with date of diagnosis or date last follow up are not required. Consequently, these have been removed:

Patient Number	FU (Years)	Outcome
10	0.45	Lost to FU
3	1.35	**Died**
9	1.46	Alive
7	1.62	Lost to FU
6	1.95	**Died**
8	1.95	Alive
2	2.34	**Died**
5	2.36	Lost to FU
4	3.12	Alive
1	4.04	Alive

Next, we give every patient a ***rank number***. We start with rank 0 and in doing so we create ***one extra row*** in the table:

Patient Number	FU (Years)	Outcome	Rank Number
			0
10	0.45	Lost to FU	1
3	1.35	**Died**	2
9	1.46	Alive	3
7	1.62	Lost to FU	4
6	1.95	**Died**	5
8	1.95	Alive	6
2	2.34	**Died**	7
5	2.36	Lost to FU	8
4	3.12	Alive	9
1	4.04	Alive	10

Next, we create an extra column where we indicate how many patients are *at risk*. We start with rank 0, were 10 patients are at risk.

The patient with rank number 1 had the shortest follow up, 0.45 years. After this time, there were 9 patients left. The next patient had a follow up of 1.35 years and died. After this event there were 8 patients left, and so on.

This is indicated in the 5th column of the table:

Patient Number	FU (Years)	Outcome	Rank Number	At Risk
			0	10
10	0.45	Lost to FU	1	9
3	1.35	**Died**	2	8
9	1.46	Alive	3	7
7	1.62	Lost to FU	4	6
6	1.95	**Died**	5	5
8	1.95	Alive	6	4
2	2.34	**Died**	7	3
5	2.36	Lost to FU	8	2
4	3.12	Alive	9	1
1	4.04	Alive	10	0

Next, we calculate the probability of failure (death). We always start with rank number 1.

The patient with rank number 1 was lost to follow up (censored) after 0.45 years. We know that the patient was alive at that time. The probability of death for this patient is 0 out of 10 patients (0/10) equals 0; leaving 9 patients at risk.

The patient with rank number 2 died after a follow up of 1.35 years. So, the probability of death in the period between 0.45 and 1.35 years is 1 out of 9 patients (1/9 = 0.1111); leaving 8 patients at risk.

The next patient was alive after a follow up period of 1.46 years. The probability of death for this patient was 0/8 (=0); leaving 7 patients at risk.

The patient with rank number 4 was lost to follow up after 1.62 years. The risk of death in the period between 1.46 and 1.62 years is therefore 0 out of 6 (=0); leaving 6 patients at risk.

125

There were 2 patients who had a follow up of 1.95 years. One of these patients died and one patient was alive. The risk of death between 1.62 and 1.95 years of follow up is therefore 1 out of 6 (=0.16667); leaving 4 patients at risk.

The next patient died after a follow up period of 2.34 years. In the follow up period between 1.95 and 2.34 years, the risk of death was 1/4 (=0.25). This left only 3 patients at risk. And so on.

The probability of death is indicated in the 6th column of the table below:

Patient Number	FU (Years)	Outcome	Rank Number	At Risk	Probability of Death
			0	10	0
10	0.45	Lost to FU	1	9	0
3	1.35	**Died**	2	8	$\frac{1}{9}$
9	1.46	Alive	3	7	0
7	1.62	Lost to FU	4	6	0
6	1.95	**Died**	5	5	$\frac{1}{6}$
8	1.95	Alive	6	4	0
2	2.34	**Died**	7	3	$\frac{1}{4}$
5	2.36	Lost to FU	8	2	0
4	3.12	Alive	9	1	0
1	4.04	Alive	10	0	0

The probability of death in all **censored** patients is 0. Therefore, the probability of death has only to be calculated in the **uncensored** patients, were the event of interest (death) occurred.

The probability of survival is 1 minus the probability of death. This has been indicated in the 7th column of the table:

Patient Number	FU (Years)	Outcome	Rank Number	At Risk	Probability of Death	Probability of Survival
			0	10	0	1
10	0.45	Lost to FU	1	9	0	1
3	1.35	**Died**	2	8	$\frac{1}{9}$	$\frac{8}{9}$
9	1.46	Alive	3	7	0	1
7	1.62	Lost to FU	4	6	0	1
6	1.95	**Died**	5	5	$\frac{1}{6}$	$\frac{5}{6}$
8	1.95	Alive	6	4	0	1
2	2.34	**Died**	7	3	$\frac{1}{4}$	$\frac{3}{4}$
5	2.36	Lost to FU	8	2	0	1
4	3.12	Alive	9	1	0	1
1	4.04	Alive	10	0	0	1

We have now calculated the probability of death from 0 to 0.45 years, 0.45 to 1.35 years, 1.35 to 1.46 years, 1.46 to 1.62 years, 1.62 to 1.95 years, 1.95 to 2.34 years and so on.

However, the probability of surviving from 0 to 1.35 years depends on first having survived from 0 to 0.45 years and than from 0.45 to 1.35 years. As explained in chapter 2, we will have to **multiply** these probabilities. Therefore, we will need to calculate the cumulative survival.

So, the probability of surviving to 1.35 years equals $1 * \frac{8}{9}$. Similarly, the

probability of surviving to 1.46 years is $1 * \frac{8}{9} * 1$ and so on.

The cumulative survival has been calculated for all patients and is indicated in the last column of the table below:

Patient Number	FU (Years)	Outcome	Rank Number	At Risk	Probability of Death	Probability of Survival	Cumulative Survival
			0	10	0	1	1
10	0.45	Lost to FU	1	9	0	1	1
3	1.35	**Died**	2	8	$\frac{1}{9}$	$\frac{8}{9}$	$\frac{8}{9}$
9	1.46	Alive	3	7	0	1	$\frac{8}{9}$
7	1.62	Lost to FU	4	6	0	1	$\frac{8}{9}$
6	1.95	**Died**	5	5	$\frac{1}{6}$	$\frac{5}{6}$	$\frac{8}{9}*\frac{5}{6}$
8	1.95	Alive	6	4	0	1	$\frac{8}{9}*\frac{5}{6}$
2	2.34	**Died**	7	3	$\frac{1}{4}$	$\frac{3}{4}$	$\frac{8}{9}*\frac{5}{6}*\frac{3}{4}$
5	2.36	Lost to FU	8	2	0	1	$\frac{8}{9}*\frac{5}{6}*\frac{3}{4}$
4	3.12	Alive	9	1	0	1	$\frac{8}{9}*\frac{5}{6}*\frac{3}{4}$
1	4.04	Alive	10	0	0	1	$\frac{8}{9}*\frac{5}{6}*\frac{3}{4}$

Or, calculated:

Patient Number	FU (Years)	Outcome	Rank Number	At Risk	Probability of Death	Probability of Survival	Cumulative Survival
			0	10	0	1	**1**
10	0.45	Lost to FU	1	9	0	1	**1**
3	1.35	**Died**	2	8	$\dfrac{1}{9}$	$\dfrac{8}{9}$	**0.8889**
9	1.46	Alive	3	7	0	1	**0.8889**
7	1.62	Lost to FU	4	6	0	1	**0.8889**
6	1.95	**Died**	5	5	$\dfrac{1}{6}$	$\dfrac{5}{6}$	**0.7407**
8	1.95	Alive	6	4	0	1	**0.7407**
2	2.34	**Died**	7	3	$\dfrac{1}{4}$	$\dfrac{3}{4}$	**0.5555**
5	2.36	Lost to FU	8	2	0	1	**0.5555**
4	3.12	Alive	9	1	0	1	**0.5555**
1	4.04	Alive	10	0	0	1	**0.5555**

Or in percentages:

Patient Number	FU (Years)	Outcome	Rank Number	At Risk	Probability of Death	Probability of Survival	Cumulative Survival (%)
			0	10	0	1	**100**
10	0.45	Lost to FU	1	9	0	1	**100**
3	1.35	**Died**	2	8	$\dfrac{1}{9}$	$\dfrac{8}{9}$	**88.9**
9	1.46	Alive	3	7	0	1	**88.9**
7	1.62	Lost to FU	4	6	0	1	**88.9**
6	1.95	**Died**	5	5	$\dfrac{1}{6}$	$\dfrac{5}{6}$	**74.1**
8	1.95	Alive	6	4	0	1	**74.1**
2	2.34	**Died**	7	3	$\dfrac{1}{4}$	$\dfrac{3}{4}$	**55.6**
5	2.36	Lost to FU	8	2	0	1	**55.6**
4	3.12	Alive	9	1	0	1	**55.6**
1	4.04	Alive	10	0	0	1	**55.6**

The 5-year cumulative survival estimated by the Kaplan-Meier method is thus 55.6%. This is very similar to the 52.4% 5-year survival as estimated by the life table method.

As in the life table analysis, we can also construct a survival curve. The survival curve in our example is as follows:

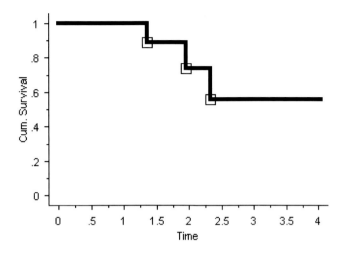

In Kaplan-Meier survival analysis, the curve is also stepped (as it is in life table analysis). However, the steps are at the times the event of interest (death) has occurred and NOT at yearly intervals. If there are many of these events, the curve will become smooth.

An example of a smooth curve is shown in the graph below. This graph shows the cumulative survival, as estimated with the Kaplan-Meier method, of patients who were diagnosed with bony metastases following a cancer:

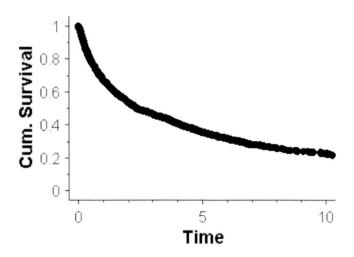

It has to be realised that the survival curve on its own does not provide all the information. One can easily be left with a false impression. It is always better to look at the table as well as the graph.

In our previous example the 5-year survival was 52.4% as estimated by life table analysis (***best-case scenario***). However, from the table it can be seen that there was only 1 patient who had a survival of more than 4 years. This patient keeps the cumulative survival at 52.4 % in the following years until he or she dies. Once the patient dies, the cumulative survival will drop suddenly from 52.4% to 0%. It might well have been that this 1 patient was wrongly diagnosed with cancer or, for reasons not completely understood, did extremely well.

So let us assume, (in our example) that this patient would live to 9.1 years instead of 4.04 years. This would change the life table as follows:

Year	FU (Years)	No @ Start	Withdrawn (Censored)	Died (Failure)	At Risk	Prob of Failure	Prob of Survival	Cumulative Survival (%)
1	>0 & ≤1	10	1	0	9.5	0	1	1
2	>1 & ≤ 2	9	3	2	7.5	$\frac{2}{7.5}$	$\frac{5.5}{7.5}$	73.3
3	>2 & ≤ 3	4	1	1	3.5	$\frac{1}{3.5}$	$\frac{2.5}{3.5}$	52.4
4	>3 & ≤ 4	2	1	0	1.5	0	1	52.4
5	>4 & ≤ 5	1	0	0	1	0	1	52.4
6	>5 & ≤ 6	1	0	0	1	0	1	52.4
7	>6 & ≤ 7	1	0	0	1	0	1	52.4
8	>7 & ≤ 8	1	0	0	1	0	1	52.4
9	>8 & ≤ 9	1	0	0	1	0	1	52.4
10	>9 & ≤ 10	1	0	1	1	1	0	0
11	>10 & ≤ 11	0	0	0	0	0		

It can be seen that the cumulative survival remains 52.4% until year 9. In year 10, it suddenly drops to 0%. This is because there was only 1 patient followed up between 4 and 10 years. This 1 remaining patient keeps the cumulative survival artificially high and gives us a wrong impression.

One has to be very suspicious when examining survival curves. It is very important to watch the 'tail end' of the curve.

Particularly suspicious are sudden large drops in the curve. This could mean that either, there were a number of patients who all failed at the same time or, more likely, that the number of patients is small and one failure caused the large drop.

The 'tail end' of the survival curve can give a wrong impression if number of patients remaining in follow up is low. It is always advisable to look at a survival curve in conjunction with the corresponding table.

For people reading publications, it is preferable to look at a graph that contains all the information. It can be very helpful to indicate the number of patients remaining in follow up next to the data points in the survival curve. If the number of patients remaining in follow up is low, the curve has to be interpreted with caution.

Another way of indicating the degree of caution one has to have in interpreting a survival curve is to calculate the 95% confidence interval. Error bars can be indicated in the survival curve. If the error bars are wide, the curve has to be interpreted with caution. There are several methods of calculating the 95% confidence interval. However, this is beyond the scope of this book.

There are two definitions that are commonly used in the literature. These are **5-year survival** and **median survival**.

5-Year Survival

The five-year survival is the cumulative probability of being alive after 5 years. This is shown in the graph below:

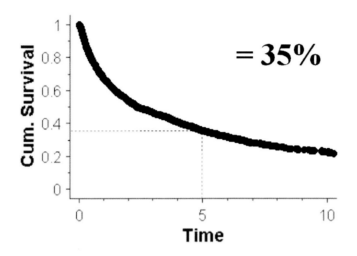

Median Survival

The median survival is the time it takes for the cumulative survival to be 50%. The graph below shows the median survival to be 2.25 years:

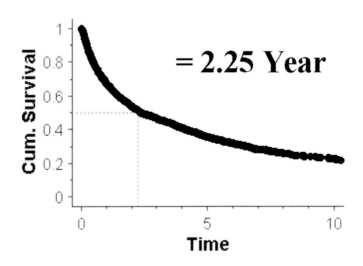

The use of survival analysis has been extended beyond estimating survival rates in cancer patients. It has also been used to estimate the survival of total joint replacements. In this case, it is not so easy to define a 'hard end point'.

In our example we have used death as an 'end point'. Death is a 'hard end point' as there is no confusion about it.

If one wants to use survival curves to estimate the longevity of total joint replacements, an 'end point' has to be chosen that indicates when the joint replacement has failed. It seems obvious to take the date the primary joint replacement has been revised to the next joint replacement as 'hard end point'. Indeed, 'revision' of the primary prosthesis is commonly used as point of failure in the published literature (see also question 10,11 & 12).

However, one has to realise that 'revision' is NOT a 'hard end point'. A surgeon might well decide not to revise an implant as the procedure is felt to be too difficult. Consequently, the patient is being counted as a 'success', whilst in reality the joint replacement has failed.

Summary Chapter 9

- Survival analysis calculates the probability of survival of a group of patients between two events, the start date and the end date

- In survival analysis it is essential to define a 'hard end point' for the event of interest

- There are several methods to perform survival analysis

- The most elementary method is life table survival analysis
  Another method is Kaplan-Meier survival analysis

- Patients are called *uncensored* if the event of interest has occurred

- Patients are *censored* if they are withdrawn from follow up

- In life table analysis, *censored* patients are at risk of the event of interest for only part of that year

- *Censored* patients are either lost to follow up, or the event of interest has not yet occurred

- **The survival curve is stepped at yearly intervals in life table survival analysis**

- **In Kaplan-Meier survival analysis, the curve is also stepped. However, the steps are at the times the event of interest has occurred. If there are many of these events, the curve will become smooth.**

- **The 'tail end' of the survival curve can give a wrong impression if number of patients remaining in follow up is low**

- **The five-year survival is the cumulative probability of being alive after 5 years**

- **The median survival is the time it takes for the cumulative survival to be 50%**

Questions Chapter 9

The table below shows 20 patients who have been diagnosed with cancer. The first column shows the follow up (in years) of the patients who were alive at review. In the second column, the follow up till time of death is indicated. The third column shows the time to last review in the patients who were lost to follow up:

Alive (Years)	Dead (Years)	Lost to Follow Up (Years)
0.2	0.6	0.8
0.4	1.2	1.4
1.5	1.4	1.8
2.2	1.9	2.1
2.5	2.1	3.6
3.1	2.5	
3.5	3.8	
4.1		

1. Calculate the 5-year survival in the **best-case scenario,** using life table analysis.
2. Calculate the 5-year survival in the **worst-case scenario,** using life table analysis.
3. Show the **best-case scenario** and **worst-case scenario** survival curves in 1 graph, using life table analysis.
4. Perform the Kaplan-Meier survival analysis in the **best-case scenario**.
5. What is the survival in Q4 at 4.1 years?
6. What is the median survival in Q4?
7. Perform the Kaplan-Meier survival analysis in the **worst-case scenario**.
8. What is the survival in Q7 at 4.1 years?
9. What is the median survival in Q7?

The table below shows the follow up data of 20 patients who had a total ankle replacement:

Number	FU (Years)	Outcome
1	1.1	Well
2	1.2	**Revised (infection)**
3	1.9	Well
4	2.1	Well
5	2.9	Well
6	3.1	Well
7	3.9	Well
8	5.0	Well
9	5.3	**Revised (aseptic loosening)**
10	5.5	Well
11	6.1	*Lost to FU*
12	6.3	Well
13	6.9	**Revised (aseptic loosening)**
14	7.1	Well
15	7.3	*Lost to FU*
16	7.4	*Lost to FU*
17	7.5	*Lost to FU*
18	8.9	Well
19	9.5	*Lost to FU*
20	10.2	Well

10. Calculate the 10-year Kaplan-Meier survival of the prosthesis using revision for *aseptic loosening* as 'hard end point'.

11. Calculate the 10-year Kaplan-Meier survival of the prosthesis using revision as 'hard end point'.

12. Calculate the 10-year **worst-case scenario** Kaplan-Meier survival of the prosthesis using revision as 'hard end point'.

Chapter 10 – Bias & Randomisation

Bias is similar to accuracy in that it observes the variation from the true value. Often however we are uncertain about the true value. This makes assessment of bias difficult.
Obviously, if the accuracy is 100%, there is no bias (unbiased).

There are many types of bias described, but they can be separated into three main groups.
- **Selection bias**
- **Confounding bias**
- **Observational bias**

Selection Bias

Selection bias occurs when there are differences between the study groups.
For example, an orthopaedic surgeon measures time to fracture healing in two groups of patients with tibial fractures. One group is treated by external fixation and the other by intramedullary nailing. If the surgeon selects the treatment method, it is likely the two groups are not comparable.
Perhaps the external fixator group contains mostly patients who had open fractures and the intramedullary nailing group patients with closed tibial fractures following football injuries. Obviously, as the groups are not comparable, this could have an effect on the outcome of the study.

Selection bias can be reduced by randomisation. For example the surgeon can, when a patient with a tibial fracture is admitted to hospital, randomise the treatment to either intramedullary nailing or external fixation. The randomisation process (rather than the surgeon) decides what treatment the patient will receive.

Confounding Bias

This really is a special form of selection bias.
We observe this form of bias when another factor (than the measured variable) influences the outcome. The factor causing the confounding bias is called the **confounding factor**.
For example, we know that smoking has adverse effect on fracture healing. Suppose, in a trial, we compare two types of osteotomy and use the time to fracture healing as the outcome measure. It could well be that there are more smokers in the one group than in the other. Obviously, this would influence the outcome of the trial. In this example, smoking is the confounding factor.
When we know something is a confounding factor, **stratification can be used to reduce confounding bias**. Stratification is a special form of randomisation. The mathematics of which is beyond the scope of this book. However, suffice to say that the stratification process assertains there are the same proportion of smokers in each study group.

Observational Bias

Observational bias is observed when there is error in measurement of disease or misclassification.
For example, this can occur when we compare the results of conservative and operatively treated tibial fractures. The fact that patients in one group had an operation whilst the other group had not; can lead to observational bias. Patients might think they are better off (or perhaps worse off) because they had an operation. Also, in assessing the outcome, the surgeon might be influenced by the fact that the patient had an operation rather than conservative treatment. This is more likely if the surgeon performed the operation him or her self.

One way of trying to reduce this bias is by requesting another surgeon to measure the outcome. However, this does not eliminate bias.
The bias could be 'in favour' or 'against' the surgical procedure.
An orthopaedic registrar performing the measurements for his / her consultant is unlikely to 'upset the boss' and therefore also biased.

Another way to ***reduce observational bias is by blinding***. Ideally the subject of investigation as well as the person measuring the outcome are blinded. This is called ***double blinding***. Obviously, this is not always possible in orthopaedics. Often, the radiographs show what procedure has been performed. In which case we will have to suffice with single blinding (if possible).

If we are dealing with animal experiments, we could perform a ***sham operation*** to try to reduce observational bias. A sham operation is an operation in the control group; the surgical exposure is the same, but no procedure is performed. Obviously, this is unethical in human studies. A sham operation is the surgical equivalent of a placebo (non functional drug given to the control group).

Another type of observational bias occurs when we measure the outcome of hip replacement with a functional scoring system (such as the Harris hip score). Such scoring systems assess pain, function and range of motion. I have already expressed my concerns relating to these scoring systems previously (chapter 5)
However, function is often assessed as walking with a frame, crutch, stick or unaided. It could well be that the patient's hip is functioning extremely well, but that the patient is walking with a stick because there is also severe arthritis in the knee. In this case, the outcome measure is not measuring what it supposed to measure (function of the hip replacement). The observational bias so introduced, can be reduced by trying to improve upon the outcome measure.

Summary Chapter 10

Bias
- **Selection bias**
- **Confounding bias**
- **Observational bias**

Randomisation reduces selection bias

Stratification reduces confounding bias

Blinding reduces observational bias

Chapter 11 – Studies & Trials

There are two types of Studies, observational studies and clinical trials.

Observational Study

These can be divided in three groups:
- **Cross sectional study**
- **Case control study**
- **Cohort study**

Cross Sectional (Prevalence) Study

A cross sectional study is also called a prevalence study. It is performed on the population that has survived. Therefore, it is prone to selection bias. Cross sectional studies are often performed in epidemiology and can be helpful in trying to establish causes for disease. For example the relation between smoking and lung cancer can be established with a cross sectional study.

Case Control Study

A case control study is a retrospective study. Patients are selected by past exposure of a risk factor and compared to a group that has not been exposed to this risk factor. Again, being retrospective, this type of study is prone to selection bias. Advantages of case control studies are that they are cheap, quick and easy to perform.
For example, suppose we suspect that smoking adversely affects fracture healing. From our records, we could identify a group of patients with tibial fractures and determine whether fracture healing is prolonged in patients who smoke.

It can be difficult selecting an appropriate control group that is similar in all but the risk factor.

An alternative case control study is where we try to match a control to each patient in the study group. The control will be similar in all (age, sex etc) but the past expose to the risk factor. This is called a case matched study. In this type of study, the control group is more comparable to the study group.

Cohort Study

A cohort study is prospective in design. A group of patients, who have been exposed to a risk factor, are followed in time and the outcome is observed. Clearly, compared to a case control study, a cohort study is more difficult to do and time consuming. It also involves considerable administration.

Another problem with cohort studies is that there is bias due to patients lost to follow up. An advantage is that the design is prospective and clearly the weight of evidence is greater as compared to a case control study (see later).

For example, we could perform a hip replacement on a group of people and follow the outcome in time.

Randomised Controlled Trial

The gold standard is the double blind randomised controlled trial. It has two arms: a study group and a control group.

As discussed in the previous chapter (chapter 10), blinding is designed to reduce observational bias and randomisation to reduce selection bias.

The advantages of a randomised controlled trial are:

- ◆ Evaluation of single variable
- ◆ Prospective study
- ◆ Reduces bias
- ◆ Allows for meta-analysis by combining several randomised controlled trials

Power Analysis

Power analysis is performed in order to determine the number of patients required in a study to demonstrate a statistically significant difference. We mentioned the power of a statistical test previously (chapters 5 & 6).
The exact mathematics is beyond the scope of this book. Also, it depends on what type of statistical analysis will be performed. However, in order to estimate the sample size we require an estimate of:

- **Difference desired to detect**
    Difference in mean (parametric)
    Difference in mode (non parametric)
- **Spread of Data**
    Standard deviation or variance (parametric)
    Range (non parametric)
- **Significance level (α)**
- **Test statistic (power)**

Steps in setting up Randomised Controlled Trial

The following steps are required in setting up a randomised controlled trial:

- **Hypothesis**
    Null hypothesis: there is no difference as opposed to the alternate hypothesis (there is a difference)

- **Inclusion / Exclusion Criteria**
    Describe the criteria for exclusion and inclusion in the study

- **Outcome Measure**
    Select outcome measure and the type of data.
    Data could be nominal, ordinal or continuous.
    Depending or the type of data, a test statistic is selected.
    If continuous data are normally distributed, parametric statistics (t-test) can be used. Alternatively, we can use a non parametric statistical test.

- **Bias**
  Assessment of bias:
  There could be selection bias, confounding bias or observational bias.
  Selection bias is reduced by randomisation.
  If there is a known confounding factor, stratification can be used to reduce confounding bias.
  Observational bias is reduced by blinding.

- **Power Analysis**
  Power analysis is performed to estimate the number of patients required in the study. It is necessary to have an estimate of:
  > *Difference desired to detect*
  > *Spread of data*
  > *Significance level*
  > *Test statistic (power)*

  A pilot study might be required to estimate these parameters.

- **Ethical Approval**

- **Informed Consent**

- **Collection of Data & Results**

- **Analysis**
  Use either parametric or non parametric tests.
  Usually computers are used in the analysis.

- **Conclusions**

- **Publication and Presentation of Data**

Hierarchy of Evidence

If the outcome of a randomised controlled trial suggests something, we are more likely to take notice than if it were published in a case report. The **weight of evidence** of a randomised controlled trial is larger than that of a case report. There is hierarchy of evidence.

The hierarchy of evidence is as follows:

Case report

Cross sectional study

Case control study

Cohort study

Randomised controlled trial

Systematic review & meta-analysis

Summary Chapter 11

Observational studies

- **Cross sectional study (prevalence)**
- **Case control study**
- **Cohort study**

Advantages of randomised controlled trial

- **Evaluation of single variable**
- **Prospective study**
- **Reduces bias**
- **Allows for meta-analysis**

Power analysis

- **Difference desired to detect**
- **Spread of data**
- **Significance level (α)**
- **Test statistic (power)**

Hierarchy of evidence

- **Case report**
- **Cross sectional study**
- **Case control study**
- **Cohort study**
- **Randomised controlled trial**
- **Systematic review & meta-analysis**

Literature

Bland M,
An Introduction to Medical Statistics
Oxford Medical Publications, 1994

Chapter 2, Survival Curves
Page 21 – 51

Nijdam B
Statistiek en Kansrekening
Tweede druk
Instituut voor Ontwikkeling van het Wiskundig Onderwijs, 1976

Szabo RM
Principles of Epidemiology for the Orthopaedic Surgeon
J Bone Joint Surgery, 80-A: 111-120, 1998

Freedman KB, Bernstein J
Sample Size and Statistical Power in Clinical Orthopaedic Research
J Bone Joint Surgery, 81-A: 1454-1460, 1998

Greenhalgh T
How to Read a Paper
BMJ Publishing Group, 1997

Answers Chapter 1

1. There were 1000 people with osteosarcoma and the population at risk was 50 million. So:

$$\text{Prevalence} = \frac{1000}{50000000} = \frac{20}{1000000} = \textbf{20 per million}$$

2. At the start of the year there were 1000 cases of osteosarcoma. 200 new cases were diagnosed and 75 patients with osteosarcoma died. On 1st January 2001 there were therefore:

1000 + 200 − 75 = 1125

patients with osteosarcoma. So:

$$\text{Prevalence} = \frac{1125}{50000000} = \frac{22.5}{1000000} = \textbf{22.5 per million}$$

3. There were 200 new cases of osteosarcoma in the year. The Incidence is therefore:

$$\text{Incidence} = \frac{200}{50000000} = \frac{4}{1000000} = \textbf{4 per million}$$

4. The two by two table is as follows:

	Disease (Kienböck's)	No Disease (No Kienböck's)
Exposure (Neg Ulnar Var)	12	138
No Exposure (No Neg Ulnar Var)	3	347

5. The relative risk is:

$$\text{Absolute Risk 1} = \frac{12}{150} = 0.08$$

$$\text{Absolute Risk 2} = \frac{3}{350} \approx 0.00857$$

$$\text{Relative Risk} = \frac{\frac{12}{150}}{\frac{3}{350}} \approx 9.33$$

6. The odds ration is:

$$\text{Odds Ratio} = \frac{12 * 347}{138 * 3} = \frac{4164}{414} \approx 10.06$$

Answers Chapter 2

1. Obviously, we need to use:

Probability $(X) = \binom{t}{n} * (c)^n * (1-c)^{t-n}$

In this case, $t = 10$, $n = 3$ and $c = 1/10$.

So:

Probability $= \binom{10}{3} * \left(\frac{1}{10}\right)^3 * \left(\frac{9}{10}\right)^{10-3} = \frac{10!}{7!*3!} * \frac{1^3}{10^3} * \frac{9^7}{10^7} = \frac{10!}{7!*3!} * \frac{9^7}{10^{10}} =$

$$\frac{10*9*8}{3*2*1} * \frac{9^7}{10^{10}} = \frac{3443737680}{6000000000\,0} \approx 0.0574 \approx 5.7\%$$

2. The total number of combinations is:
We start by painting 9 of the 20 objects red.

There are $\binom{20}{9}$ possible combinations of doing that.

Of the remaining 11 objects, we paint 8 white. That can be done in $\binom{11}{8}$ possible combinations.

The final three objects are painted blue. Obviously there is only one possible combination of doing that.
The total number of possible combinations is thus:

$$\binom{20}{9} * \binom{20-9}{8} * \binom{20-9-8}{3} = \binom{20}{9} * \binom{11}{8} * \binom{3}{3} = \frac{20!}{11!*9!} * \frac{11!}{3!*8!} * \frac{3!}{3!} =$$

$$\frac{20!}{9!} * \frac{1}{3!*8!} = \frac{20*19*18*17*16*15*14*13*12*11*10}{3*2*1*8*7*6*5*4*3*2*1} =$$

27713400

One might think that the answer would have been different if we would have started by painting the 3 blue objects. The following formula describes the possible combinations by first painting 3 objects blue, followed by 8 objects white:

$$\binom{20}{3} * \binom{20-3}{8} * \binom{20-3-8}{9} = \binom{20}{3} * \binom{17}{8} * \binom{9}{9} =$$

$$\frac{20!}{17!*3!} * \frac{17!}{9!*8!} * \frac{9!}{9!} = \frac{20!}{3!} * \frac{1}{8!} * \frac{1}{9!} = 27713400$$

Indeed, if we would have started by painting the 8 white objects, followed by nine objects red, the formula would have been:

$$\binom{20}{8} * \binom{20-8}{9} * \binom{20-8-9}{3} = \binom{20}{8} * \binom{12}{9} * \binom{3}{3} =$$

$$\frac{20!}{12!*8!} * \frac{12!}{3!*9!} * \frac{3!}{3!} = \frac{20!}{8!} * \frac{1}{9!} * \frac{1}{3!} = 27713400$$

So, it doesn't make any difference where you start. We have shown that:

$$\binom{20}{9} * \binom{11}{8} * \binom{3}{3} = \binom{20}{3} * \binom{17}{8} * \binom{9}{9} = \binom{20}{8} * \binom{12}{9} * \binom{3}{3}$$

3. This is very similar to the example given in the main text. The probability is:

$$\frac{\binom{4}{1} * \binom{1}{1} * \binom{3}{2} * \binom{44}{1}}{\binom{52}{5}} = \frac{\dfrac{4!}{3!*1!} * 1 * \dfrac{3!}{1!*2!} * \dfrac{44!}{43!*1!}}{\dfrac{52!}{47!*5!}} = \frac{4!*3!*44!*47!*5!}{3!*2!*43!*52!} =$$

$$\frac{47!*44!*5!*4!*3!}{52!*43!*3!*2!} = \frac{44*5*4*3*4*3*2}{52*51*50*49*48} = \frac{70560}{311875200} \approx 0.000226$$

4. $$\frac{\binom{4}{1}*\binom{1}{1}*\binom{3}{0}*\binom{44}{3}}{\binom{52}{5}} = \frac{\frac{4!}{3!*1!}*1*1*\frac{44!}{41!*3!}}{\frac{52!}{47!*5!}} = \frac{4!*44!*47!*5!}{3!*1!*41!*3!*52!} =$$

$$\frac{47!*44!*5!*4!}{52!*41!*3!*3!} = \frac{44*43*42*5*4*4}{52*51*50*49*48} = \frac{6357120}{311875200} \approx 0.0204 \approx 2\%$$

5. This probability can be calculated by adding the probability of 1 king plus the probability on two kings plus the probability on three kings plus the probability of four kings:

$$\text{Probability} = \frac{\binom{4}{1}*\binom{48}{4}}{\binom{52}{5}} + \frac{\binom{4}{2}*\binom{48}{3}}{\binom{52}{5}} + \frac{\binom{4}{3}*\binom{48}{2}}{\binom{52}{5}} + \frac{\binom{4}{4}*\binom{48}{1}}{\binom{52}{5}} =$$

$$\frac{\frac{4!}{3!*1!}*\frac{48!}{44!*4!}}{\frac{52!}{47!*5!}} + \frac{\frac{4!}{2!*2!}*\frac{48!}{45!*3!}}{\frac{52!}{47!*5!}} + \frac{\frac{4!}{1!*3!}*\frac{48!}{46!*2!}}{\frac{52!}{47!*5!}} + \frac{1*\frac{48!}{47!*1!}}{\frac{52!}{47!*5!}} =$$

$$\frac{\frac{4!}{3!*1!}*\frac{48!}{44!*4!} + \frac{4!}{2!*2!}*\frac{48!}{45!*3!} + \frac{4!}{1!*3!}*\frac{48!}{46!*2!} + \frac{48!}{47!*1!}}{\frac{52!}{47!*5!}} =$$

$$\frac{\frac{48!}{44!*3!} + \frac{48!}{45!} + \frac{48!*2}{46!} + \frac{48!}{47!}}{\frac{52!}{47!*5!}} =$$

$$\frac{\frac{48*47*46*45}{3*2} + \frac{48*47*46}{1} + \frac{48*47*2}{1} + \frac{48}{1}}{\frac{52!}{47!*5!}} =$$

$$\frac{8 * 47 * 46 * 45 + 48 * 47 * 46 + 48 * 47 * 2 + 48}{\left(\dfrac{52 * 51 * 50 * 49 * 48}{5 * 4 * 3 * 2}\right)} =$$

$$\frac{886656}{2598960} \approx 0.34158$$

It would have been simpler to calculate the probability that no king is drawn and subtracting this from 1:

$$\text{Probability} = 1 - \frac{\binom{4}{0} * \binom{48}{5}}{\binom{52}{5}} = 1 - \left(\frac{1 * \dfrac{48!}{43! * 5!}}{\dfrac{52!}{47! * 5!}}\right) = 1 - \left(\frac{48!}{43! * 5!} * \frac{47! * 5!}{52!}\right) =$$

$$1 - \left(\frac{48! * 47! * 5!}{52! * 43! * 5!}\right) = 1 - \left(\frac{48! * 47!}{52! * 43!}\right) = 1 - \left(\frac{47 * 46 * 45 * 44}{52 * 51 * 50 * 49}\right) =$$

$$1 - \left(\frac{4280760}{6497400}\right) \approx 1 - 0.659 \approx 0.341158$$

6. $$\text{Probability} = \frac{\binom{6}{6} * \binom{43}{0}}{\binom{49}{6}} = \frac{1}{\left(\dfrac{49!}{43! * 6!}\right)} = \frac{1}{\left(\dfrac{49 * 48 * 47 * 46 * 45 * 44}{6 * 5 * 4 * 3 * 2}\right)} =$$

$$\frac{1}{\left(\dfrac{49 * 48 * 47 * 46 * 45 * 44}{6 * 5 * 4 * 3 * 2}\right)} \approx 0.0000000715$$

Answers Chapter 5

1. Using <= 16 weeks as 'cut off' point, we indicate patients were fracture healing had occurred within 16 weeks by '-'. Patients who took longer than 16 weeks to unite their fracture are indicated by '+':

Patient	Group	Time to Fracture Healing (Weeks)	Sign
1	Smoker	10	-
2	Smoker	11	-
3	Smoker	11	-
4	Smoker	12	-
5	Smoker	15	-
6	Smoker	17	+
7	Smoker	17	+
8	Smoker	18	+
9	Smoker	18	+
10	Smoker	19	+
11	Smoker	22	+
12	Smoker	24	+
13	Non Smoker	10	-
14	Non Smoker	10	-
15	Non Smoker	11	-
16	Non Smoker	12	-
17	Non Smoker	15	-
18	Non Smoker	15	-
19	Non Smoker	16	-
20	Non Smoker	17	+

In the smoking group, there were 7 out of 12 patients were fracture union was in excess of 16 weeks. Whilst In the non smokers, there was only 1 out of 8 patients were the fracture took longer than 16 weeks to unite. Is this due to chance?

We formulate a null hypothesis; *there is no difference in fracture healing time between smokers and non smokers* and test this hypothesis.

Using a **two sided** sign test the probability is:

$$P = \binom{8}{1} * (0.5)^1 * (0.5)^7 + \binom{8}{0} * (0.5)^0 * (0.5)^8 +$$

$$\binom{8}{7} * (0.5)^7 * (0.5)^1 + \binom{8}{8} * (0.5)^8 * (0.5)^0$$

$$P = \frac{8!}{7! * 1!} * (0.5) * (0.5)^7 + \frac{8!}{8! * 0!} * (0.5)^8 +$$

$$\frac{8!}{1! * 7!} * (0.5)^7 * (0.5) + \frac{8!}{0! * 8!} * (0.5)^8$$

$$P = 8 * 0.00390625 + 1 * 0.00390625 +$$
$$8 * 0.00390625 + 1 * 0.00390625$$

$$P = 0.0703125$$

$P > 5\%$, therefore NOT statistically significant.
The null hypothesis can therefore NOT be rejected. We conclude that we were unable to demonstrate a difference in fracture healing time between smokers and non smokers.

2. Using the Chi Square test, we need to first construct a table with the observed frequencies:

	Smoker	Non Smoker	Total
<= 16 weeks	5	7	12
> 16 weeks	7	1	8
Total	12	8	**20**

Next we calculate the expected frequencies:

	Smoker *Observed*	Smoker *Expected*	Non Smoker *Observed*	Non Smoker *Expected*	Total
<= 16 weeks	5	12*12/20	7	8*12/20	12
> 16 weeks	7	12*8/20	1	8*820	8
Total	12		8		**20**

	Smoker *Observed*	Smoker *Expected*	Non Smoker *Observed*	Non Smoker *Expected*	Total
<= 16 weeks	5	7.2	7	4.8	12
> 16 weeks	7	4.8	1	3.2	8
Total	12	12	8	8	**20**

Using the Chi Square test statistic:

$$\sum \frac{(O-E)^2}{E}$$ (O = Observed frequency and E = Expected frequency)

$$\sum \frac{(O-E)^2}{E} = \frac{(5-7.2)^2}{7.2} + \frac{(7-4.8)^2}{4.8} + \frac{(7-4.8)^2}{4.8} + \frac{(1-3.2)^2}{3.2}$$

$\approx 0.6722 + 1.00833 + 1.00833 + 1.5125$

≈ 4.2014

The observed frequency table has two rows and two columns. There is therefore 1 degree of freedom (r-1)*(c-1). Using the Chi Square distribution table we can see that there is statistical significance (p< 5%).

The above question shows that statistical significance can be demonstrated using the Chi Square test, but not the sign test. The Chi Square test is therefore a *more powerful* test than the sign test.

Answers Chapter 7

1.   First we construct a table:

	Truth *positive*	**Truth** *negative*	
Test *positive*	6	4	10
Test *negative*	30	10	40
	36	14	**50**

True Positive:	6
False Positive:	4
False Negative:	30
True Negative:	10

Positive Predictive Value: $\dfrac{6}{10}$ = 60%

Negative Predictive Value: $\dfrac{10}{40}$ = 25%

Sensitivity: $\dfrac{6}{36}$ ≈ 17%

Specificity: $\dfrac{10}{14}$ ≈ 71%

Accuracy: $\dfrac{16}{50}$ = 32%

2.   No

Answers Chapter 8

1.
    a.
    b.

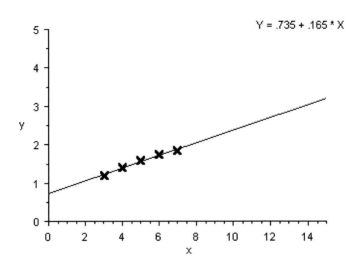

c. The computer calculated:
      y = 0.735 + 0.165*x (using the least square method)

If estimated:

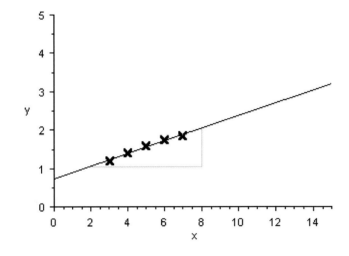

b = 0.75

$$a = \frac{\Delta y}{\Delta x} = \frac{2-1}{8-2} = \frac{1}{6} = 0.167$$

So: y = 0.75 + 0.167*x

2. The line fits the data extremely well. Therefore, the correlation coefficient should be close to 1.
   The computer calculated:
   $r^2 = 0.983$
   So,
   $r = \sqrt{0.983} = 0.991$

3. If we substitute x = 5.5 in
   $y = 0.735 + 0.165*x$
   $y = 0.735 + 0.165 * 5.5$
   $y = 0.735 + 0.9075$
   $y = 1.6425$

4. If we substitute x = 0.1 in
   $y = 0.735 + 0.165*x$
   $y = 0.735 + 0.165 * 0.1 = 0.7515$
   If we substitute x = 15 in
   $y = 0.735 + 0.165*x$
   $y = 0.735 + 0.165 * 15 = 3.21$

5. The computer plotted the data points of the extended data set and fitted the best curve using the least square method. The equation of the curve is given in the graph.

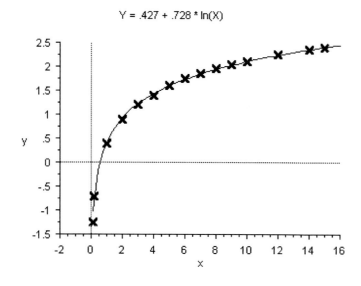

6. X and y have a logarithmic relation. The correlation coefficient is extremely close to 1.

7. We can look up the y-values for x = 0.1 and x = 15 in the table.

X	Y
0.1	**-1.25**
0.2	-0.7
1	0.4
2	0.9
3	1.2
4	1.4
5	1.6
6	1.75
7	1.85
8	1.95
9	2.05
10	2.1
12	2.25
14	2.35
15	**2.4**

Alternatively, one can substitute them in the found formula:
y = 0.427 + 0.728 * Ln(x)

For x = 0.1
y = 0.427 + 0.728 * Ln(0.1)
y = -1.25

For x = 15
y = 0.427 + 0.728 * Ln(15)
y = 2.4

One can see that these values are very different from the ones found in question 4. This question illustrates again the danger of extrapolating data!

Answers Chapter 9

For convenience, the table is shown below:

Alive (Years)	Dead (Years)	Lost to Follow Up (Years)
0.2	0.6	0.8
0.4	1.2	1.4
1.5	1.4	1.8
2.2	1.9	2.1
2.5	2.1	3.6
3.1	2.5	
3.5	3.8	
4.1		

1. The **best-case scenario** life table is as follows:

Year	FU (Years)	No @ Start	Withdrawn (Censored)	Died (Failure)	At Risk	Prob of Failure	Prob of Survival	Cumulative Survival (%)
1	>0 & ≤1	20	3	1	18.5	$\dfrac{1}{18.5}$	$\dfrac{17.5}{18.5}$	94.6
2	>1 & ≤ 2	16	3	3	14.5	$\dfrac{3}{14.5}$	$\dfrac{11.5}{14.5}$	75.0
3	>2 & ≤ 3	10	3	2	8.5	$\dfrac{2}{8.5}$	$\dfrac{6.5}{8.5}$	57.4
4	>3 & ≤ 4	5	3	1	3.5	$\dfrac{1}{3.5}$	$\dfrac{2.5}{3.5}$	41.0
5	>4 & ≤ 5	1	1	0	0.5	0	1	41.0

So, the 5-year survival in the *best-case scenario* as estimated with life table analysis is 41%.

2. The ***worst-case scenario*** life table is as follows:

Year	FU (Years)	No @ Start	Withdrawn (Censored)	Died (Failure)	At Risk	Prob of Failure	Prob of Survival	Cumulative Survival (%)
1	>0 & ≤1	20	2	2	19	$\dfrac{2}{19}$	$\dfrac{17}{19}$	89.5
2	>1 & ≤2	16	1	5	15.5	$\dfrac{5}{15.5}$	$\dfrac{10.5}{15.5}$	60.6
3	>2 & ≤3	10	2	3	9	$\dfrac{3}{9}$	$\dfrac{6}{9}$	40.4
4	>3 & ≤4	5	2	2	4	$\dfrac{2}{4}$	$\dfrac{2}{4}$	20.2
5	>4 & ≤5	1	1	0	0.5	0	1	20.2

So, the 5-year survival in the *worst-case scenario* as estimated with life table analysis is 20%.

3. Using the tables constructed in Q2 and Q3, we can plot the survival curves in a graph:

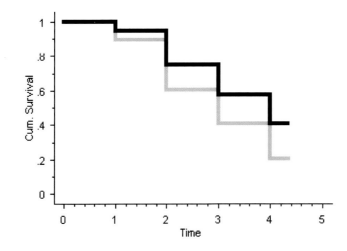

The ***best-case scenario*** is shown in black and the ***worst-case scenario*** is shown in grey.

4. In the ***best-case scenario***, the patients lost to follow up count as a success. The Kaplan-Meier table is as follows:

Rank Number	FU (Years)	Outcome	At Risk	Probability of Death	Probability of Survival	Cumulative Survival (%)
0			20			**1**
1	0.2	Alive	19	0	1	**1**
2	0.4	Alive	18	0	1	**1**
3	0.6	**Died**	17	$\dfrac{1}{18}$	$\dfrac{17}{18}$	**94.4**
4	0.8	*Lost to FU*	16	0	1	**94.4**
5	1.2	**Died**	15	$\dfrac{1}{16}$	$\dfrac{15}{16}$	**88.5**
6	1.4	**Died**	14	$\dfrac{1}{15}$	$\dfrac{14}{15}$	**82.6**
7	1.4	*Lost to FU*	13	0	1	**82.6**
8	1.5	Alive	12	0	1	**82.6**
9	1.8	*Lost to FU*	11	0	1	**82.6**
10	1.9	**Died**	10	$\dfrac{1}{11}$	$\dfrac{10}{11}$	**75.1**
11	2.1	**Died**	9	$\dfrac{1}{10}$	$\dfrac{9}{10}$	**67.6**
12	2.1	*Lost to FU*	8	0	1	**67.6**
13	2.2	Alive	7	0	1	**67.6**
14	2.5	**Died**	6	$\dfrac{1}{6}$	$\dfrac{5}{6}$	**56.3**
15	2.5	Alive	5	0	1	**56.3**
16	3.1	Alive	4	0	1	**56.3**
17	3.5	Alive	3	0	1	**56.3**
18	3.6	*Lost to FU*	2	0	1	**56.3**

19	3.8	**Died**	1	$\frac{1}{2}$	$\frac{1}{2}$	**28.2**
20	4.1	Alive	0	0	1	**28.2**

5. **The survival at 4.1 years in the *best-case scenario* as estimated with Kaplan-Meier analysis is 28%.**

6.   For the answer to this question we need to plot the survival curve:

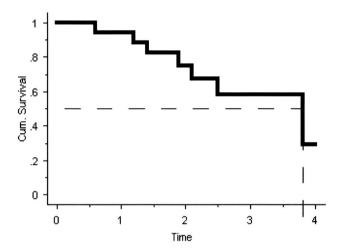

It can be seen from the graph that the median survival ≈ 3.75 years.

7. In the ***worst-case scenario***, the patients lost to follow up count as a failure. The Kaplan-Meier table is as follows:

Rank Number	FU (Years)	Outcome	At Risk	Probability of Death	Probability of Survival	Cumulative Survival (%)
0			20			1
1	0.2	Alive	19	0	1	1
2	0.4	Alive	18	0	1	1
3	0.6	**Died**	17	$\dfrac{1}{18}$	$\dfrac{17}{18}$	94.4
4	0.8	*Lost to FU*	16	$\dfrac{1}{17}$	$\dfrac{16}{17}$	88.9
5	1.2	**Died**	15	$\dfrac{1}{16}$	$\dfrac{15}{16}$	83.3
6	1.4	**Died**	14	$\dfrac{1}{15}$	$\dfrac{14}{15}$	77.8
7	1.4	*Lost to FU*	13	$\dfrac{1}{14}$	$\dfrac{13}{14}$	72.2
8	1.5	Alive	12	0	1	72.2
9	1.8	*Lost to FU*	11	$\dfrac{1}{12}$	$\dfrac{11}{12}$	66.2
10	1.9	**Died**	10	$\dfrac{1}{11}$	$\dfrac{10}{11}$	60.2
11	2.1	**Died**	9	$\dfrac{1}{10}$	$\dfrac{9}{10}$	54.2
12	2.1	*Lost to FU*	8	$\dfrac{1}{9}$	$\dfrac{8}{9}$	48.1
13	2.2	Alive	7	0	1	48.1
14	2.5	**Died**	6	$\dfrac{1}{7}$	$\dfrac{6}{7}$	41.3
15	2.5	Alive	5	0	1	41.3
16	3.1	Alive	4	0	1	41.3

17	3.5	Alive	3	0	1	**41.3**
18	3.6	*Lost to FU*	2	$\frac{1}{3}$	$\frac{2}{3}$	27.5
19	3.8	**Died**	1	$\frac{1}{2}$	$\frac{1}{2}$	13.8
20	4.1	Alive	0	0	1	13.8

8. **The survival at 4.1 years in the *worst-case scenario* as estimated with Kaplan-Meier analysis is 14%.**

9. For the answer to this question we need to plot the survival curve:

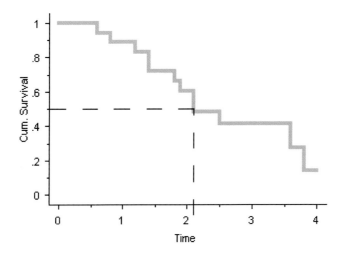

One can see from the graph that the median survival ≈ 2.25 years.

10. Only patients who had a 'Revision' for ***aseptic loosening*** are counted as failures. The Kaplan-Meier table is as follows:

Rank Number	FU (Years)	Outcome	Outcome	At Risk	Probability of Failure	Probability of Survival	Cumulative Survival (%)
0				20			
1	1.1	Well	Success	19	0	1	100
2	1.2	Revised (infection)	Success	18	0	1	100
3	1.9	Well	Success	17	0	1	100
4	2.1	Well	Success	16	0	1	100
5	2.9	Well	Success	15	0	1	100
6	3.1	Well	Success	14	0	1	100
7	3.9	Well	Success	13	0	1	100
8	5.0	Well	Success	12	0	1	100
9	5.3	Revised (aseptic loosening)	Failed	11	$\dfrac{1}{12}$	$\dfrac{11}{12}$	91.7
10	5.5	Well	Success	10	0	1	91.7
11	6.1	Lost to FU	Success	9	0	1	91.7
12	6.3	Well	Success	8	0	1	91.7
13	6.9	Revised (aseptic loosening)	Failed	7	$\dfrac{1}{8}$	$\dfrac{7}{8}$	80.2
14	7.1	Well	Success	6	0	1	80.2
15	7.3	Lost to FU	Success	5	0	1	80.2
16	7.4	Lost to FU	Success	4	0	1	80.2
17	7.5	Lost to FU	Success	3	0	1	80.2
18	8.9	Well	Success	2	0	1	80.2
19	9.5	Lost to FU	Success	1	0	1	80.2
20	10.2	Well	Success	0	0	1	80.2

The 10-year Kaplan-Meier survival for aseptic loosening is therefore 80%:

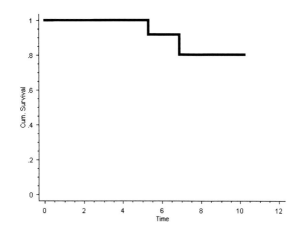

11.   All patients who had a 'Revision' are counted as failures. The Kaplan-Meier table is as follows:

Rank Number	FU (Years)	Outcome	Outcome	At Risk	Probability of Failure	Probability of Survival	Cumulative Survival (%)
0				20			
1	1.1	Well	Success	19	0	1	100
2	1.2	Revised (infection)	Failed	18	$\dfrac{1}{19}$	$\dfrac{18}{19}$	94.7
3	1.9	Well	Success	17	0	1	94.7
4	2.1	Well	Success	16	0	1	94.7
5	2.9	Well	Success	15	0	1	94.7
6	3.1	Well	Success	14	0	1	94.7
7	3.9	Well	Success	13	0	1	94.7
8	5.0	Well	Success	12	0	1	94.7
9	5.3	Revised (aseptic loosening)	Failed	11	$\dfrac{1}{12}$	$\dfrac{11}{12}$	86.8
10	5.5	Well	Success	10	0	1	86.8
11	6.1	*Lost to FU*	Success	9	0	1	86.8
12	6.3	Well	Success	8	0	1	86.8
13	6.9	Revised (aseptic loosening)	Failed	7	$\dfrac{1}{8}$	$\dfrac{7}{8}$	76.0
14	7.1	Well	Success	6	0	1	76.0
15	7.3	*Lost to FU*	Success	5	0	1	76.0
16	7.4	*Lost to FU*	Success	4	0	1	76.0
17	7.5	*Lost to FU*	Success	3	0	1	76.0
18	8.9	Well	Success	2	0	1	76.0
19	9.5	*Lost to FU*	Success	1	0	1	76.0
20	10.2	Well	Success	0	0	1	76.0

The 10-year Kaplan-Meier survival for revision is therefore 76%:

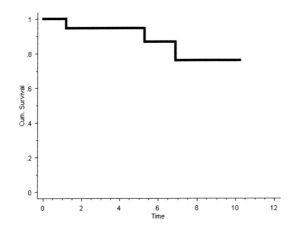

12. In the ***worst-case scenario***, all patients who are lost to follow up are also counted as a failure:

Rank Number	FU (Years)	Outcome	Outcome	At Risk	Probability of Failure	Probability of Survival	Cumulative Survival (%)
0				20			
1	1.1	Well	Success	19	0	1	100
2	1.2	**Revised (infection)**	**Failed**	18	$\dfrac{1}{19}$	$\dfrac{18}{19}$	94.7
3	1.9	Well	Success	17	0	1	94.7
4	2.1	Well	Success	16	0	1	94.7
5	2.9	Well	Success	15	0	1	94.7
6	3.1	Well	Success	14	0	1	94.7
7	3.9	Well	Success	13	0	1	94.7
8	5.0	Well	Success	12	0	1	94.7
9	5.3	**Revised (aseptic loosening)**	**Failed**	11	$\dfrac{1}{12}$	$\dfrac{11}{12}$	86.8
10	5.5	Well	Success	10	0	1	86.8
11	6.1	*Lost to FU*	**Failed**	9	$\dfrac{1}{10}$	$\dfrac{9}{10}$	78.2
12	6.3	Well	Success	8	0	1	78.2
13	6.9	**Revised (aseptic loosening)**	**Failed**	7	$\dfrac{1}{8}$	$\dfrac{7}{8}$	68.4
14	7.1	Well	Success	6	0	1	68.4
15	7.3	*Lost to FU*	**Failed**	5	$\dfrac{1}{6}$	$\dfrac{5}{6}$	57.0
16	7.4	*Lost to FU*	**Failed**	4	$\dfrac{1}{5}$	$\dfrac{4}{5}$	45.6
17	7.5	*Lost to FU*	**Failed**	3	$\dfrac{1}{4}$	$\dfrac{3}{4}$	34.2
18	8.9	Well	Success	2	0	1	34.2
19	9.5	*Lost to FU*	**Failed**	1	$\dfrac{1}{2}$	$\dfrac{1}{2}$	17.1
20	10.2	Well	Success	0	0	1	17.1

The *worst-case scenario* 10-year Kaplan-Meier survival for revision is therefore 17%:

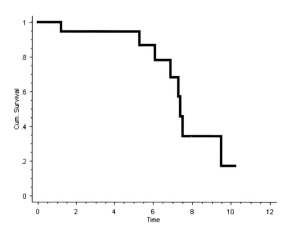

These questions illustrate the importance of choosing a 'hard end point'. They also show that if all patients lost to follow up are counted as a failure (***worst-case scenario***), the survival curve drops steeply.

There was not much difference in the 10-year survival for 'revision' and 'revision for aseptic loosening'. This is because the one patient who had an infection had this relatively early (at 1.2 years). At this time there were 18 patients who had a longer follow up. Consequently, the effect on the failure rate (1 out of 19) is not as big as it would have been if only 1 patient had a longer follow up (1 out of 2).
So, a failure at the 'tail end' (longer follow up) of the survival curve has a far more pronounced effect on the cumulative survival than a failure at the beginning (short follow up).